Incurable
LUNGS

If you, a friend, caregiver, spouse, or family member are dealing with a devastating disease, this book is intended to provide a story of lessons learned and a message of hope.

Life will get better.

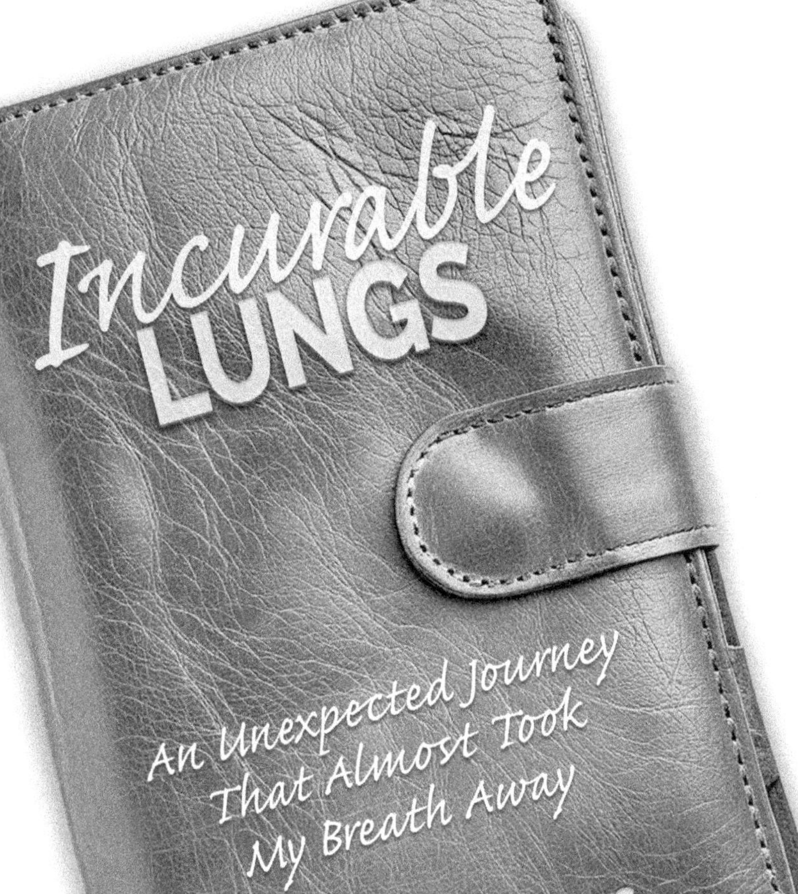

Thomas Williams

Incurable LUNGS

An Unexpected Journey That Almost Took My Breath Away

© 2024 Thomas Williams

All rights reserved. No portion of this book may be reproduced, stored in a retrieval system, or transmitted in any form or by any means—electronic, mechanical, photocopy, recording, scanning, or other—except for brief quotations in critical reviews or articles, without the prior written permission of the publisher.

Inquiries regarding permission for use of the material contained in this book should be addressed to: twilliams@incurablelungs.com

ISBN: 979-8-218-50751-0

The net proceeds from this book will go to the Pulmonary Fibrosis Foundation and Donate Life Kentucky.

Copy Editor: Kathleen Pothier, Positively Proofed, info@positivelyproofed.com

Cover and Interior Design: Melissa Farr, Back Porch Creative, LLC,
Melissa@backporchcreative.com

Contents

Preface

This book is a collection of short stories about surviving an incurable interstitial lung disease (ILD). Some of the stories were written at different times along my journey, and some were from before I even knew I had the disease. These scenarios helped me address the challenges of ILD. To put my thoughts at that time into perspective, each entry is dated. (All entries have been edited for clarity and brevity.)

The Pulmonary Fibrosis Foundation (pulmonaryfibrosis.org) and the United Network for Organ Sharing (unos.org) have been a tremendous help to me and many others with lung diseases, as well as their caregivers.

There is a growing number of organ transplants in the U.S. each year, with more than 42,000 overall. However, there are fewer than 3,000 lung transplants—and about 85% of those recipients survive the first year. The waiting list and times vary depending on donors and other factors. While the list and number of transplants grow, there are, unfortunately, thousands wanting to qualify to get on this list. My wait, once I qualified, was seven months, with two nerve-racking dry runs. Some only wait for a week, while others wait for as long as two years. The system to match donors and candidates is complicated and is currently being revised, which may help the process. Waiting for a transplant while keeping in shape in order to survive is very stressful. Many on the list, unfortunately, do not make it before they get the call.

There are more than 150,000 people diagnosed in the United States each year with my disease, Idiopathic Pulmonary Fibrosis (IPF), and nearly a million others have other critical ILD where a transplant may eventually be their best option. This staggering statistic was hard for me to grasp when applying to get on the list. How could I have been so fortunate as to become one of these recipients?

While there is no known cause of IPF, nor is there a cure, there is ongoing research to identify the causes (or triggers), as well as new medications to delay the progression. They are very expensive and have side effects. My research leads me to believe that a combination of two or more factors—including but not limited to genetic, environmental, health factors, medications for other health problems, and exposures to toxins—are major contributors. My research also makes me believe that environmental and air-quality factors cause the disease to progress more rapidly. This impacted our decision to move out of Houston after my diagnosis.

Writing the following short stories has helped me better understand how all this happened, how I was able to survive, and why it is always good to have a "Plan B." I have kept a daily diary for many years, which was helpful to document some of the challenges, as well as the fun I have had along the way. I hope others with my disease will do the same.

The most important factors in my recovery have been family, friends, faith, and determination. It would have been impossible for me to have made it this far without the excellent medical care I received at the University of Kentucky Transplant Center in Lexington, Kentucky.

Donating an organ is a generous act that will outlive you for many generations to come. Just go to organdonor.gov to learn more.

Introduction

This book is a compilation of my stories. From these experiences, I learned how to survive complications caused by a life-changing illness. The more we learn and communicate with others, the better we will all get through it. I appreciate life in a different way, as I am sure all transplant recipients do. We all wish we did not belong to this club, but we are willing to help those in it.

Once I made it to Year Two—through a round of COVID and a few setbacks—I was noticeably getting stronger, both physically and mentally. The visits to the doctor are less frequent but still necessary. I have a long way to go, and I realize life is never easy, but choosing to enjoy life is a blast.

It has been great moving back to Central Kentucky—where it is not too hilly, not too flat, and as close of a place to heaven as I have found. There are few places better than Keeneland in April and October. I love the Gulf Coast and its salty air, but I can't think of a better place where bourbon, horses, basketball, good music, and religion are properly intertwined. Unlike anywhere else, the people I have met throughout my travels who left Kentucky to pursue their careers still consider themselves Kentuckians, and most wish to someday return home. My IPF disease caused me to return sooner than I had planned and, unfortunately, not soon enough to spend time with my parents before they died.

In some ways, this disease was not all a bad thing. If anyone who faces their own certain mortality "sooner than later" is not motivated to get one's life in order, nothing else can. It causes you to figure out what is important. When bad things like this happen, we all have to decide upon our own definition of "quality of life" going forward, but we also need to live to the fullest and make our own choices. They are ours to make, not our doctors'.

These stories explain my choices. Writing them down was intended to help others deal with making their own choices, but this has also been a therapeutic blessing to me. Thanks to my new lungs and gift-of-life miracle, I now have more time. I have been so lucky to be able to celebrate true joy with my wife, Gale.

Chapter One

How a Friend's Lung Transplant Changed My Life

My journal writings in August 2020

Sixteen years ago, I received a call from Bob Gentile, a friend I worked for at the U.S. Department of Energy (DOE) in Washington, D.C., in the early '90s. He wanted me to know that Bobby Dolence, a former colleague, had recently contracted an aggressive lung infection and needed a double-lung transplant to survive. Bob said the diagnosis was "not good," but he lived near Pittsburgh, where the University of Pittsburgh Medical Center had an excellent pulmonary and organ-transplant program. He said he would keep me informed on his progress and then gave me his address.

Bobby is about my age, a bright guy, a hard worker with a good family and a promising future back in his home state of Pennsylvania. He worked with Bob, who was then the director of the Office of Surface Mining at the U.S. Department of Interior during the Reagan administration, and we met when I worked for Bob at the DOE. We were not close but just friends who shared common beliefs and values. I was not able to reach Bobby by phone. I can't explain it, and I had not spoken to him in a few years, but his news hit me pretty hard. I did not know much about lung transplants other than they were rare and risky.

I was living in Houston, achieving professional success in the oil and gas business while working long hours and traveling a lot, yet I had little extra time for myself or my family. I had recently missed spending quality time with my dad before he died of liver cancer, and I saw little of my family back in Kentucky or my best fishing buddy in Florida. I grew up fishing with my dad and we spent countless hours together on the water. I can't believe I thought work was too important to take time off. I was frustrated because my priorities had become "out of sorts."

The next morning, I took off work to buy Bobby a get-well card and a book—*A Salty Piece of Land* by Jimmy Buffett—which I had recently enjoyed because it had taken my mind off my day-to-day stresses. I included a note telling him he would be as good as new once he got his new lungs and could then go on an adventure like the character in the book, Tully Mars.

This was well before the era of Google when the library and bookstore were the best sources of information. At the bookstore that morning I also learned a little about transplants and how there's a shortage of people willing to be organ donors. I found out I could be a donor by signing my driver's license, which I did for the first time. I also found another book, *Chasing Daylight* by Eugene O'Kelly, described as an inspirational read about a successful CEO dealing with a terminal illness. I have no idea how I stumbled on that book, but it seemed appropriate to include in the package I planned to mail the next day. That night, I was still thinking about my friend and started reading the book I bought for Bobby. I continued to read until I finished it before the next morning. It was awesome and life changing.

That moment in time was a tipping point for me because I realized I needed to make some major changes in my life. The news about how a healthy friend all of a sudden may not make it caused me to think about life's "what ifs," especially since I had had a few near misses in my life. This was the first time I had a sense of urgency, and I was determined to make changes.

Bobby had a successful transplant; he is healthy today and volunteers at the University of Pittsburgh Medical Center (UPMC) transplant and patient programs. He also sits on the advisory board to the Center for Organ Recovery and Education (CORE). He is totally unaware about how his illness ended up changing my life.

Thanks to Bobby's transplant and the book, my life eventually got a whole lot better: It was not easy, but more fulfilling, albeit a work in progress. I think that is the way it is supposed to be.

I could have never imagined what was in store for me in the future and how it could possibly be related to this moment.

In 2018, Gale and I were living and working in Houston, and we had recently sold our weekend house in Matagorda on the Texas coast. We moved our fishing boat to a marina in Rockport, where we would visit about once a month, and we were finally taking some nice trips. I tried to semi-retire, but I had been pulled back to work in the oil and gas business as president of high-profile, not-for-profit organization Research Partnership to Secure Energy for America (RPSEA).

My new job required a lot of travel, and I noticed I was becoming progressively out of breath and tired. At Gale's insistence, I visited my family doctor, who ordered some tests, including a CT. After eliminating a pulmonary embolism, she suspected I might have IPF. I was then sent to a specialist for more testing. Following the tests, a pulmonary doctor confirmed to both me and Gale that I had IPF. He said there was no cure, and the disease was progressive and terminal. He told us that a lung transplant might eventually be an option. At that point, his words were going in one ear and out the other.

How could this have happened? My life was good; I was happy. I was taking time to enjoy life more—travel, bike ride, and go fishing. We sold our weekend house on the Texas coast to free up our time to travel.

Ironically, Gale had accepted a job in Lexington, Kentucky, just a few months before my symptoms were apparent. Her new job was with Ledcor, a large, diversified company based in Canada, with operations in Kentucky. It was a nice opportunity for Gale because Ledcor was a good company to work for, and they were growing. Lexington is near our family and a very nice place to live. Fortunately, after my diagnosis, they provided us with excellent health insurance.

After Gale accepted her new job, we purchased a 125-year-old house in the historic section of downtown. The house needed a lot of renovation, but at that time we had no idea what was about to happen. We had planned to split time between Houston and Lexington until I retired. I thought I might do some consulting, but mostly enjoy life. I thought perhaps we would buy a winter home in Florida near my best friend, Jim Toombs. However, with the IPF diagnosis, I retired as fast as practical. We eventually sold our Houston house and moved full time to Kentucky.

I began to research the disease and my options. I looked at ongoing research and clinical trials. I eventually (and fortunately) got a second opinion at the Vanderbilt Pulmonary and Transplant Center in Nashville, Tennessee. After my diagnosis, I also called my old friend Bobby, and he was a tremendous resource (and still is). He assured me that I could deal with what would come next. Bobby always stressed not to let the perfect get in the way of the good. At that time, I was willing to settle for the unknown as an alternative to the terrible.

At the recommendation of our doctor at Vanderbilt, I started pulmonary rehab and am on the lung transplant list at the University of Kentucky. I am on several prayer lists and get messages of support from friends and family all the time. This is very helpful. I am determined that once I get through this, I plan to inform others about the value of organ transplants and how to deal with life-altering challenges.

Chapter Two

Getting the Word

Written August 2021

There are probably more than a million people in the U.S. every year who are told by their doctor that they have a potentially terminal disease.

We have all read accounts of how different people take this kind of news. Many develop a new sense of urgency to get their spiritual life in order, others reflect on life's failures, or they worry about finances and prepare for the "inevitable." Others start the grieving process, while some diligently develop a plan to combat the disease. My guess is that several just wait and do what they are told to do next. Their disease could be cancer, Alzheimer's, ALS, or many others.

In my case, my family doctor in Houston sent me to a pulmonologist in early 2018 after she suspected I had a lung disease, possibly IPF. The pulmonary doctor conducted additional tests and, in a matter-of-fact diagnosis, told me and Gale that I had IPF, a disease with no known cause and no cure. At that point, the best I can remember, he said to avoid "looking it up on Google." My memory was pretty foggy at that point. My initial reaction was disbelief, but I had options.

My doctor recommended medication that might delay the disease. He said he would see me every month or so. The medication he prescribed was extremely expensive and, according to the clinical trials, did not always work and had several bad side effects. Over the course of a few months, I experienced several of those side effects, including being tired, headaches, stomach problems and, at times, flu-like symptoms. My cough continued to get worse. I convinced him to change to another equally expensive medication that was similar in reported effectiveness. These pills were about $9,000 per month! The side effects were bad but not as severe.

My disease continued to progress, and we do not know if the medication slowed the progression or not. The doctor offered few other options. I regularly rode my bike along the trails of Houston and was instructed to use an oximeter, which is a small device that helps measure the levels of oxygen in the blood. He said if my levels got below 88%, I should stop and rest, but if they got below 84%, I needed to call his office immediately. Normal healthy levels are over 95%. Taking him at his word, my bike riding was quickly over because my oxygen levels fell below 88% with any brisk exercise. I asked him about rehab or any other things I could do to improve my quality of life. He discouraged it. In hindsight, I made some poor choices by not quickly getting a second opinion and taking more control of my health.

I decided to learn everything I could about my disease and all the various options available. There was a lot of information and, particularly—once I found out where to find them—peer-reviewed papers. I eventually found valuable resources that my Houston doctor did not provide. I contacted researchers working on the cause, and I found medications to slow the progress. The Pulmonary Fibrosis Foundation was one of the better resources.

Being in the energy research business for many years and having written and read tons of technical papers was a bonus. They are not like reading a novel. The footnotes and references many times provide a map to the information you are trying to find. For anyone who has been diagnosed with a lung disease, regardless of whether you are a tenacious researcher like me or not, the PFF website is an excellent starting spot. They can also provide a lot of data, as well as a source for support groups. Connecting with other patients is also very important.

There is no one way for anyone to know how to deal with life-changing news. Balancing work, family, and normal day-to-day dealings with finances, responsibilities, feeling bad, and managing various priorities all become very complicated in a hurry. Gale's support was a tremendous help, but it became exceedingly difficult for her with a new job, an old house needing remodeling, and especially me being away in Houston. I knew I had to reprioritize my life and figure out what I had to do in order to get better (or at least not any worse), understand how this impacted Gale, and then we could make future priorities from there.

I had no time to worry or think about what may or may not happen but instead what I could do to extend my life. I recalled how a former boss once told me that to be successful in business, you need to "keep the main thing the main thing." This was sage advice during my new life crisis. It is hard to not get distracted.

This all took me a little while, but we began the process of developing a plan for how to live. While I believe no one can give you a road map on what is the right thing to do, the more questions you ask, the better chances you have of developing your best plan. Changing doctors and getting additional opinions saved my life.

All this would be awfully hard going it alone. Gale was there to help us get through this. The best advice I could ever give to those who must deal with this tragic news is to appreciate the value of the primary caregiver. It is easy to become angry. In fact, this entire process would have been almost impossible without emotional support. I am one of the lucky ones. When there is another person who will stand by you, life's decisions are a lot less stressful. The future becomes more possible.

This is when my daily corporate diary became a health journal. I documented everything that would help my doctors and my health plan. These notes allowed me to write this book.

Eventually my research led me to meeting with the head of the pulmonology department at Vanderbilt: Dr. James E. Loyd. He is an awesome and nationally respected pulmonologist. They had been doing a lot of interesting clinical trials and studies on genetic causes of my disease and new medications to slow the progression.

My favorite cousin, Nancy Dunkerly, and her husband, Bob, who was a well-respected doctor in Nashville, were a tremendous help to us. We had a place to stay and people we respected to discuss our situation. The doctors at Vandy helped us develop a plan, which included rehab, medications, supplemental oxygen, and the eventual need for a transplant.

We made several trips to Nashville and always received a good evaluation and advice. On one trip he pulled me to a private room and told me there were a lot of researchers at Vanderbilt who would love to get me on a clinical trial. He said my notes, records, and decent health made me an excellent candidate, then he said, "Go get a transplant." Wow, like your favorite uncle giving you the best advice you could ever get. He also told us about the cost and complications, so we needed to make sure our insurance was in good shape. There were some issues in coverage at some hospitals, including Vanderbilt, that convinced us to go look for our best option.

I eventually made my way to the University of Kentucky (UK) after Dr. Loyd suggested I participate in their pulmonary rehab program and explore their transplant options since we had a home in Lexington. I then met Dr. James McCormick, who was the pulmonary lead at UK. He is a caring person who was helpful to me in getting into the transplant program. That's where I met Dr. Maher Baz, who eventually became my transplant doctor. He guided me through the evaluation process, and then he would be the doctor to take over from the transplant surgeon. These are all excellent, compassionate doctors. They monitored my vitals and prescribed oxygen and medication, as well as took care of my health. Dr. McCormick would check in on me from time to time during my rehab (pre- and post-transplant) because his office was nearby.

The evaluation process is very thorough and intense. On Jan. 20, 2020, as part of the evaluation process, they found a blockage in one of my arteries, which they called "the widow-maker." So, they put in a stent. The CT the day prior did not show the problem, but the cardiac catheterization did. This delayed my transplant by a few months, but the procedure no doubt saved my life the first time.

Throughout this process I drew mental strength from my mom, who was the toughest person I have ever known. She had to deal with many significant health challenges in her life, and she took them head on. She died in May 2017.

Many times during my health crisis, I wished she was still alive, but in a way, I was also glad she did not have to see me go through this. My mother figured things out many years ago. She demonstrated throughout her life, especially when times got tough, the example of having a "strong will" to live. She knew about faith, determination, rehab, and taking the advice of good doctors. In my case, I was also fortunate to have the support of family and many good friends across the country.

Like my mom, I am motivated to continue working to get better every day, ride out the bad days, and look forward to the better ones. I am a living example of the power of prayer and the impact others can have on one's life. I have a lot to live for.

Chapter Three

Matagorda

April 2016

I recall the morning my friend Dave Burnett called me and said I needed to buy a weekend place in Matagorda, Texas. At that time, I was very busy with my job at Noble Corporation because my work responsibilities were expanding. My work also required me to participate and hold leadership roles in various energy organizations, which took a lot of time. I was achieving a successful career in the energy industry.

Dave was ten years older than me, but he exercised regularly, did not work as many hours, and he was in better shape. We ran 5Ks and 10Ks together, and he always held back his pace in order to finish the races with me. He had recently married Marian, a gal he met on a sailing cruise in the Caribbean, and he had convinced her to move from Wisconsin to Houston. I gave her a part-time consulting job working on a website in the early dot-com days.

Her landlord owned a weekend house on the Colorado River, which was a few miles upriver from Matagorda and the Gulf of Mexico. Her landlord was getting older and could not keep the property maintained, so she convinced Dave and Marian to buy the house. While driving to the beach one weekend, Dave noticed some new developments and thought one of these houses would make a good investment for me, both financially and mentally.

All I knew about Matagorda was that it's a tiny fishing village about one hundred miles from my Houston home, and I had been fishing there a couple of times with my good friend Lanny Schoeling. They hosted a big fishing tournament every year called the Texas Oilman's Charity Invitational Fishing Tournament, which raised a lot of money for charity. They had a very nice marina on the Intracoastal Waterway near this small town. That was about it.

Dave sent me the name of a local real estate agent and we arranged to meet the following weekend. It did not take me long to figure out this was the perfect place to get away.

There was a new housing development on the beach road halfway between Matagorda and the beach. Beach Road is about five miles long and follows a roughly twenty-foot-deep, one-hundred-fifty-foot-wide, man-made canal that diverts the Colorado River past the Intracoastal and locks to the Gulf of Mexico. The main river had originally run into West Matagorda Bay. This channel provided Matagorda's commercial fishing fleet easy access to the Gulf. The sports fishermen who eventually built houses along the road could easily travel to the Gulf or either of the two bays: East Matagorda Bay and the much larger West Matagorda Bay.

Back then, you had to cross an old swing bridge on the Intracoastal to get to Beach Road. The road ended at a twenty-mile-long barrier island and undeveloped public beach, which the public could drive on. There was a fishing pier, a nature center, and a campground at the end of the road. Along the way were a couple of places to eat, a bait shop, and a hundred or so houses that ranged from shacks to very nice beach homes.

There was a famous annual cattle drive where the cows were rounded up on the barrier island of West Matagorda Bay and driven across the Colorado to Beach Road. Then cowboys herded the cattle across the swing bridge to downtown Matagorda, where they were loaded up to go to market. This tradition had been going on for many years.

We had a large private dock and boat lift under an elevated deck over the river. This ended up being one of the best decisions I ever made. This became my escape home away from work and the city. Several neighbors who were from the Houston area were like an extended family that helped celebrate darn near anything worth celebrating. Gale made a lot of friends, and I tagged along. My son, Adam, and his wife, Liz, were married on the beach. Our friends had to learn to sing "My Old Kentucky Home" as the requisite for my mint juleps and Derby glasses. We called it our sleepy little drinking town with a fishing problem. Mosquitoes could be bad at times, but they were part of the deal.

I later learned that Matagorda was one of the oldest towns in Texas and an important shipping port. Novelist Louis L'Amour wrote *Matagorda*, which provided some embellished history about the post-Civil War 1800s. I found it hard to believe Matagorda had once been a thriving port but now had fewer than one thousand residents, a K-8 grade school, and the oldest Methodist and Episcopal churches in Texas, along with a few other churches. There was a post office in the same building as Stanley's, which was the only store in town. (If Stanley did not have it, you did not need it.) There is a masonic lodge in Matagorda, one of the best marinas in the state, and it's home to an active shrimp and oyster fleet.

We invited our family and friends to visit Matagorda, and I was able to master catching red fish. It turned out that Matagorda was on the map after all because it consistently won the Audubon's annual Christmas Bird Count, which brought a lot of bird watchers to the area. There was an abundance of wildlife in the area and an oversized dog named Mason, who was well-fed on the weekends and fended for himself during the week. My life continued to be much better. Matagorda was changing as well, with a new bridge to replace the swing bridge, several more houses built, and a few more small businesses and places to eat.

Our days in Matagorda ended in the evening on our deck as we toasted the sunset and watched the birds fly to their nightly destination. It was serene and peaceful. We took tons of sunset photos, as this is one of my best memories of our life together. Our dog, Colonel, just added to the joy of our family and being together.

Dave and Marian occasionally made it down, and we would take our boat up the river to visit them from time to time. We went to the Easter Sunrise Service on the beach, Adopt-A-Beach cleanups, and celebrated many holidays together. Dave ran into some bad luck as he fought off non-Hodgkin's lymphoma during this time, but he continued to work at Texas A&M University (TAMU). He credits Matagorda and MD Anderson Cancer Center in Houston with helping him recover. Life was challenging for him but, looking back, he said it was the best of times.

Dave's cancer reminded me of the sense of urgency I had after I read the *Chasing Daylight* book several years prior. He was determined to beat cancer, and he did. His dedication and optimism were an example to me. This helped me get through my challenges later on.

We learned more about our Matagorda community from our neighbors Ed and Mary Ann, who were the lone full-time residents. He was a retired superintendent of the local school and a former football coach. Gale and I enjoyed spending time with them. They even included us in their family gatherings.

One day he told us about the situation of some of the families who lived in Matagorda. Ed later introduced us to the current school superintendent, Laura Shay, who opened our eyes to the community. She explained about how this town was "the end of the road," where a lot of people escaped from society. Drugs were prevalent and many of the kids lived with one parent or grandparents.

Laura was a member of the Methodist Church, whose members started an after-school latchkey program to help the kids keep up with schoolwork, have something to eat, and stay out of trouble. Laura arranged for us to meet with the teachers and the latchkey kids. She identified some families in need from time to time, and we were always willing to provide some help. We always wanted to make sure they had a good Christmas, without knowing who we were. We also helped support the Methodist Church's food bank and other civic fundraising events. Gale and I must have stuffed over a thousand plastic Easter eggs with money and candy for their annual event.

For a small town, they had quite a few community events and festivals. Laura invited us to a school function at their new gym to see the kids perform. She came by and pointed out some of the kids whom we had helped out. She was so grateful and emotional when we showed up with stuff for the kids. But we were the ones who were grateful.

I was being pulled back to work and board commitments in Houston, so Gale decided to work as well. We had a home in Houston, but Matagorda was our home most weekends. Life commitments were forcing us to make some difficult decisions about Matagorda. We sold our weekend home and made plans to travel and explore new adventures.

Turning Sixty

Gale asked me to plan my upcoming milestone sixtieth birthday. I turned sixty on Sept. 28, 2012, and it came way too early. For my fiftieth, I ran a half marathon with Dave and my buddy Lanny and was not up for another challenge like that. I decided I wanted to spend my birthday in Matagorda. The Methodist Church allowed us to use their fellowship hall.

Gale and I celebrated in Matagorda by having a themed birthday party, and we invited all the "latchkey kids" in Matagorda. It was a grand party! After due diligence, Angry Birds it was. You have no idea how much Angry Birds stuff they make, even hats. We had an Angry Bird cake, ice cream, and punch with Angry Bird cups and plates. We all had a special time on my big 6-0. We bought a variety of birthday gifts for every kid and played games until each one had won at least one nice birthday gift.

The Methodist Church annex served as the home to the latchkey program. It is the oldest Methodist church west of the Mississippi. The old building has survived hurricanes and hard times quite well. The teachers of the program were also invited to the party because they were remarkable. They did what I consider "the Lord's work" in helping the kids in the community, providing them with a place to go after school, a healthy snack and mentoring, and helping with their homework. They had strong support from the community, but they depended on donations.

Gale and I helped out when we heard they were short on supplies, computers, snacks, or whatever we heard they needed. The program is well-supported by the community. Matagorda has limited financial means, and many of the kids were being raised by grandparents or one parent. The fishermen, oystermen and shrimpers, lived pretty hard lives, and the kids paid the price. They could not help the situation they were in. This community-supported program gave them a shot to get ahead. In return, they all gave me a fine way to turn sixty.

Finally, family and friends called that birthday night to wish me a Happy Birthday. They probably thought I had lost my mind when we told them about the party. I believed it would be hard to top when I turned seventy.

I had no idea what was in store. In hindsight, ten years later, this was quite an understatement!

Turning Seventy

After surviving my lung transplant and a pretty tough COVID isolation period, I considered turning seventy a miracle. I thought I had made it over the roughest part, but rejection could come at any time. My immunity was almost nonexistent, but I wanted to get out and see things. I was not sure how effective wearing a mask was, but at least it could not hurt. I wanted to spend my seventieth birthday fishing with my best friend, Jim, on my boat in Florida. A year earlier, such an event was far from certain. Jim has a larger offshore fishing boat, and the plan was for him to use my bay boat any time he wanted and to keep it running. We would then plan our next big adventure when my doctors gave me the green light.

I was apprehensive about flying, wanting to avoid airports and crowds for the next few years, so I decided to buy myself a travel van for my birthday gift. I found one at a Winnebago dealer in Louisville that was just the right size. Gale and I started making plans for some exciting road adventures. We bought the van and two days later were on the road to the Toombs' home in St. Pete Beach, Florida, just a couple of days before my birthday. We had a big party planned with his family and some of my cousins, who lived on the east coast of Florida.

But all good plans are sometimes not meant to be! Along comes a warning for hurricane Ian. It was headed our way, so right after we arrived, our job was to help secure their home and head inland because it was projected to hit Tampa Bay. Gale and I rode out two bad hurricanes in Texas, so we were more mentally prepared than our friends.

The van came in handy to hold supplies from their home in case the worst happened. The decision was to go inland to Orlando and stay in a condo they were able to secure for us. It took a while to get there because others were also leaving the storm's path and the roads were jammed. We cleaned out their refrigerator, ate well, and celebrated my big day through a bad wind and rainstorm in Orlando. The wrath of Ian went south and destroyed the area around Fort Myers Beach, but their home and the St. Pete area were not significantly damaged. We celebrated my birthday with cake and a glass of Blanton's Bourbon. It was a birthday I will never forget.

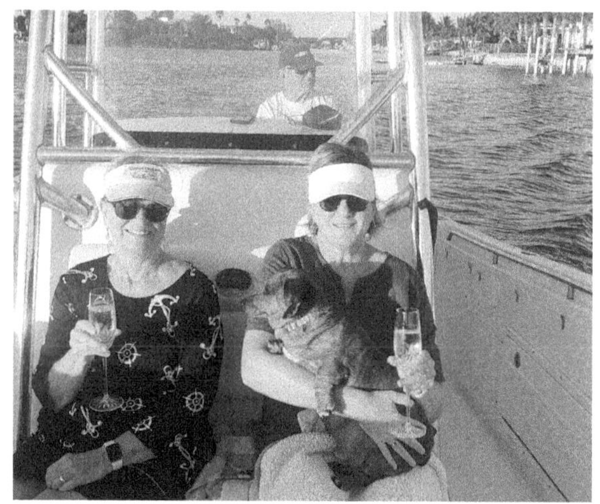

Boat Drinks 2019
A great day to be alive.

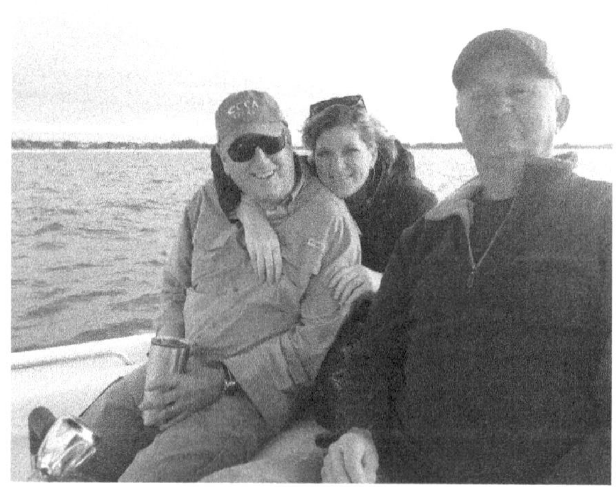

Jim, Gale, and Tom returning from fishing.

Chapter Four

Wrapping Up a Career

October 2021

I had a ringside seat in the energy business, starting in the mid-1980s. I was in the oil and gas business in Kentucky when on a business trip to Washington—through a lot of coincidences and help from my lifelong friend Kelly Sinclair, who worked in the presidential personnel office—I was offered a job at the Department of Energy (DOE) working for the George H.W. Bush administration. I knew it was a good enough opportunity for me and my family to sell my company and move. At the time, I did not know how much.

There were several of my Kentucky college friends who had moved to Washington, D.C., during the Reagan administration. I knew there would be a good network of Kentucky friends at our new home, which would make the transition easier.

Charlie Grizzle, my friend from Kentucky who was working at the Environmental Protection Agency (EPA), insisted I go to government charm school so I could learn the rules and keep out of trouble. That was great advice. I found Washington to be a strange world of smart, well-educated people, but few had real-world, practical experience. There were a few exceptions, fortunately. It takes a lot to navigate this environment. It is a competitive place as well. This experience was preparing me for future challenges I could have never anticipated.

In 1993, after the end of the H.W. Bush administration, I was offered some interesting jobs, but my priority was to work in the energy business, which meant I needed to move to Houston.

My life takes a turn in 2018

The energy business is the driver of our economy and almost everything we do. What an honor for a kid from a small town in Kentucky to have experienced it the way I did. I met many people who went out of their way to help me succeed.

In looking back at my career, one may say I could not hold down a good job. I worked for some great organizations. Some were large organizations, and some were start-ups. Each job brought new opportunities and challenges I thoroughly enjoyed. I worked with some of the best and brightest people in our country. My former boss at Noble Corp. was Jim Day. He was one of the best and a role model. My work allowed me to travel all across the U.S. and visit many countries while working on some very interesting projects.

My goal as I got older was to slow down while serving on a few corporate and not-for-profit boards and do a little consulting.

Life was too short to continue to work all the time, I told myself. However, in 2016 I was offered a job for RPSEA, a not-for-profit research consortium that I previously helped get started and had previously served on their board of directors. They were funding some good research, so I decided to take the offer. It was one of those "I knew better" decisions.

My job required a lot of traveling and attending a lot of conferences. It was challenging, and many times I wondered what I was thinking when I agreed to accept. I have always been a high-energy person, but I was not keeping up the pace I had been able to in years prior.

Then…I was diagnosed in early 2018 with IPF after a trip to Washington, D.C., with some of my board members. I became winded while walking from meeting to meeting. I knew something had been wrong for a while because I had been lacking my normal energy level, but I dismissed it as getting a little older with too little exercise. I also had a dry cough.

Back in Houston, I was fortunate that my family doctor aggressively pursued a diagnosis. I am glad Gale insisted that I go. She *strongly* insisted I go, to put it bluntly.

After some tests, I was sent by my family doctor to get a CT to eliminate the possibility of a pulmonary embolism (PE) and then to a pulmonary doctor to diagnose and confirm I had a lung disease, then to provide a prognosis. He said matter-of-factly that I had Idiopathic Pulmonary Fibrosis. I had never heard of IPF until my family doctor mentioned it. While waiting, I was afraid that I had COPD or a lung infection. Those diagnoses would have been a blessing in comparison!

The doctor had more testing done and said I would not be able to travel much and, in effect, it would be difficult to do my job for very long. He said there were some medications that would possibly slow the progression. I had an incurable lung disease and was provided some limited information. He said I should avoid high elevations like the Denver area, where I had traveled nine times the prior year. He also said to avoid believing what I read on Google. That should have been a red flag, but at the time I was not absorbing the impact of my disease. I was never told about the Pulmonary Fibrosis Foundation or other resources assisting pulmonary fibrosis patients.

Tests showed my lung capacity and blood oxygen level were decreasing rapidly. The CT and other tests confirmed "glassing" or scarring in my lungs. They give you a pulmonary function test to monitor your breathing capacity. It was hard to process. I did not have time for this! How could I break this to our members and my board? How could I break this to my friends and family?

The disease and the side effects of the medication I was prescribed to slow IPF's progression were also taking a rapid physical and mental toll. I had no choice at this point.

2018 was an important year for us. Gale was going to celebrate her fiftieth birthday. This was in September when my friend Charlie Grizzle was honored with the Henry Clay Distinguished Kentuckian Award by the Kentucky Society of Washington in Washington, D.C. Although we are both from Kentucky, D.C.

is where Gale and I met and became instant friends. We planned to attend Charlie's event, then fly to Coeur d'Alene, Idaho, to attend an Interstate Oil and Gas Compact Commission (IOGCC) meeting, and then spend a few days in Walla Walla, Washington, to visit wine country.

I was not feeling well, but I was not going to miss this trip. My IPF had not progressed to the point where I required supplemental oxygen, but I had to take it slow and monitor my oxygen levels. My cough was getting worse, and my headaches increased. This was the appropriate time to tell friends and colleagues I had worked with for years about the disease and to discuss the changes we were forced to make. It needed to be done face to face, if at all possible. This was one of the best trips I have ever taken, but in the back of my mind I thought it might be one of my last.

On the way back, Gale flew to our new home in Kentucky for her job and I headed to Houston via Denver. I had to make a quick connection and, while rushing to my gate in the airport, I ran out of air. A nice lady, who said she was a nurse, approached me and recognized my situation. The next thing I knew, I was given some oxygen. I do not recall exactly what all happened, but at the time she seemed to be an angel from heaven who was there to help me out. I quickly recovered, although I was a little shaken up. I actually made my connection and, on the flight back, I recalled my doctor's warnings about avoiding high altitudes. This was a sobering moment in my journey.

Back at work, I had mixed priorities and obligations, including the most important one to Gale and my future health. I also needed to spend a lot of time learning about the disease so I could plan out my options. Looking back, it is hard to believe how conflicted my priorities were. They should not have been.

One of my RPSEA board members whom I had known for a long time was Steve Holditch. He was the head of the petroleum engineering department at TAMU and, before that, had a successful professional career. He told me he had a heart condition. I thought he probably appreciated my situation more than most people. He came to a meeting after I announced I was leaving, pulled me aside, gave me a hug, and provided the best advice I could have had at the time. He said to just focus on my health. His insight provided an easier path going forward. This reminded me of a prior boss's advice to keep the main thing the main thing. It is easy to get distracted, even in these conditions.

Steve recently died from his heart condition and, unfortunately, I did not realize how dire his situation was. This was right after my transplant, and I had not been able to tell him I had made it. I am sure he will be one of the first I will see in heaven. I owe him a thank-you.

My quest for a successor eventually led to a former business partner, Rich Haut. It was a little painful but all in all a good transition. Rich was very capable and knew the organization well. I provided him with good documentation, records, and a clean audit so his job would not be as taxing.

Before I left, while dealing with the effects of my lung disease, I wrote a report documenting the history of the RPSEA organization and lessons learned on how to conduct a successful public-private partnership. I also made a number of presentations to various industry groups based on that report. I think it is the best document I have ever written, and I hope it will be used for future related endeavors. I am glad I fulfilled my commitments. Those presentations allowed me to see a lot of people in the industry I will never see again.

It was behind me, and now it was time to take Dr. Holditch's advice. It was hard not to look over my shoulder, however.

It is an understatement to say I had been on a steep learning curve throughout my entire career. I began an even steeper learning curve dealing with my health. My limited understanding of lung transplants from my friend Bobby and my inclination to research almost everything was a blessing to me when I was diagnosed with my disease. I believed that I had to understand the causes of my IPF and what factors may contribute to my future. It also provided a network of incredible scientists and resources.

People with terminal diseases are forced to make similar decisions, just like I had to do. No one wants to go through this, but it happens all the time. Well-run companies and leaders have a succession plan in place. Mine was done on the fly.

My outcome could have been a lot worse. I am now able to document some of the things I was able to accomplish, and I hope that others can benefit from these experiences. My daily journal has been very helpful, but it has not been easy for me to read while writing this book.

I also hope this story helps others realize what can happen in life and how a wild dream and determination can make a difference. I made plenty of mistakes along the way.

Many of my former colleagues found out about my disease and provided support during my next journey in life. The notes, prayers, and best wishes helped pull me through. The memories of working together for a worthy cause is a wonderful testament of the good in mankind.

Chapter Five

Birds, Dirt, and Sushi

January 10, 2022

Written one year and four days following my transplant and my son Adam's birthday.

Part of the orientation given to transplant patients includes a list of what to avoid and things not to eat. They provide you with a catalog, and a nutritionist meets with you and your caregiver before and after the transplant to review the list and explain what and why you can't have certain things. The anti-rejection medications elevate most people's blood sugar, which complicates your diet even more. They impact your blood pressure. They increase the risk of skin cancer, so you are told to avoid the sun. People hate to be told what they can't do or have.

The anti-rejection medications are required for the rest of your life, which means your system can't fight off infections, bad things in food like bacteria, air impurities or bad things found in dirt. Normal people have a natural immunity to these things or, at worse, healthy people may just end up with a 24-hour bug. For people like me who have new lungs while taking anti-rejection medications, these precautions are more critical for folks like me than they are for other organ recipients because the lungs are the body's first line of defense.

Needless to say, avoiding environmental pollutants and poor air quality—including dust and smoke fumes—are necessary. This also includes avoiding people who may be carrying something you can catch and put you in the hospital.

One of the medications I must take is prednisone, which is a steroid that has a lot of bad side effects, such as weight gain, diabetes, insomnia, loss of bone density, and cataracts. I call it the "devil drug." I recently had cataract surgery as a result, and I am being treated for bone density loss. I rarely get a good night's sleep.

I take about thirty pills a day, which are sometimes changed after bloodwork at the clinic. Some are needed to counteract the side effects of others. If my kidney or liver function change, they may switch my meds. Another pill, Tacrolimus, must be kept within a range to work properly. It has a long list of side effects and, coupled with all the others, they all say I am supposed to avoid the sun. My dermatologist and I are becoming buddies these days. They tell you these things up front, but until all this happens, it is hard to appreciate how powerful these medications are.

I needed to wear a mask and use hand sanitizer long before COVID came along. At least now I am in the company of others.

In my former job I learned a lot about air-quality issues, emissions, and health effects. Many lung problems are related to exposure to bad things in the air, like particulate matter. After my diagnosis, I became convinced that living in an area with good air quality will prolong my quality of life. This is one of the reasons we moved from Houston to Lexington.

The EPA publishes reports on air quality and levels of particulate matter in the air. This is something people with pulmonary fibrosis and those recovering from a lung transplant need to know but are rarely told by their doctors. Even airborne allergies become much more difficult to tolerate.

These changes are part of the lifestyle tradeoffs for all transplant patients. It is important to understand and deal with new limitations, particularly foods, from the lifestyle you previously enjoyed. One must deal with tradeoffs all the time as we determine what is our best quality of life. This is a choice I make all the time. This is not easy, but it outweighs the potential consequences. It is a choice all transplant patients and their caregivers must make.

The risk of fungal bacterial infections and viruses are the reason you have to avoid gardening and mowing the yard. You are supposed to limit indoor plants. They all can lead to infections and rejection. As cautious as I have been the first year, I had a bout of aspergillus where the symptoms were pretty bad and sent me to the hospital. It took months to get over it. The medication I was given, Voriconazole, had a number of bad side effects as well, and they were almost as bad as the infection itself.

Foods like eggs, milk, cheese, honey, juice, and cider must be pasteurized. No more raw honey. These are things I never even paid attention to before. We try to follow the temperature guidelines for food, which is 145 degrees for steaks and fish, 160 degrees for pork and eggs, and 165 degrees for chicken and deli meats. It is not easy, but we know what could happen if we don't. No more egg white in a whiskey sour? I never bothered to ask.

For people who love to cook and eat like we do, overcooking is terrible. Why bother ordering a nice steak or salmon if they are cooked to death? We are starting to adapt, learning new methods, and using our sous vide, for example, in order to get certain meats to the proper temperature and not terribly overcooked. The crockpot is also getting more use in our home.

All of a sudden, expiration labels take on new meaning and the "smell test" is no longer valid. The refrigerator and pantry are purged regularly.

These restrictions require us to check food labels closely and take added precautions, like warming cold cuts and delivered food. My staple food, in addition to hot buffalo wings, is pickled bologna. It is a Kentucky delicacy called "pickled dog," which I have eaten all my life. I never mentioned this to the nutritionist because I did not want to argue in case it was possibly off limits. I am sure she does not appreciate the nutritional value, as this is one of those great pleasures in life, just like having a good, cold beer every now and then. If it were bad for you, I would be dead by now.

I was advised to avoid certain fruits, in particular grapefruit and pomegranate. Also, ginger and turmeric should be avoided; I was never a huge fan anyway. In protest, I have decided to limit my diet by avoiding at least two green vegetables: broccoli and brussels sprouts. Actually, I have limited eating them for a long time. This just makes it official. The good news is that I need to reduce my potassium level, and spinach is one of the main culprits. Good riddance, spinach!

My doctor was adamant that I never order a salad in a restaurant because he said the risk of contamination was too high. Gale double-washes our salad greens. Our hospital nutritionist said that eating ice cream at McDonald's was a death wish. Fortunately, she is a very good person, and we seem to run into her from time to time at a local brewery. It is good to get excellent nutritional advice over a cold beer.

The things I will miss the most are raw oysters, sushi, and rare steak. When we go to the Caribbean, I do not know how I will avoid conch salad and ceviche. This reminds me of a saying my dad always told me growing up: It is "better to want what you don't have than have what you don't want." I always thought he was talking about girls, but it sure applies to this situation (I guess).

Seasonal allergies are more of a problem now, which means I need to wear a mask outside during certain times of year. Bird droppings are a big cause of fungal infections in people with no immunity. We took down the bird feeder on our deck.

I have enjoyed growing a garden all of my life, so I will miss putting plants in the ground and watching them grow. Most of our indoor plants are also gone. Gale is now in charge. When fresh mulch is being spread, I wear a mask and stay inside. Getting out of lawn mowing is not as good as it sounds.

One of my biggest concerns is air pollutants, which are almost impossible to avoid. Of particular concern to me as an avid fisherman is avoiding algae blooms, as is the case in southwest Florida, where they recently had a severe breakout of Karenia brevis, called red tide. Data show that even low levels can cause immunocompromised people to have respiratory problems and pneumonia. I used my past position as an adviser to the Gulf of Mexico Foundation to seek out some of the scientists studying red tide. They all advised me to stay clear when it is bad. I even have a red tide app, thanks to the work being done by the National Oceanic and Atmospheric Administration (NOAA) researchers and the Florida Fish and Wildlife Conservation Commission. This has caused us to rethink our long-term plans. This is where my boat is, where my best friend and his family live, and a wonderful place to live. We will need to figure this out.

Airborne mold is a big issue because my system can quickly detect it.

I am also supposed to avoid cats. I have never liked them anyway, and they cause me to sneeze. This will be an easy thing to avoid.

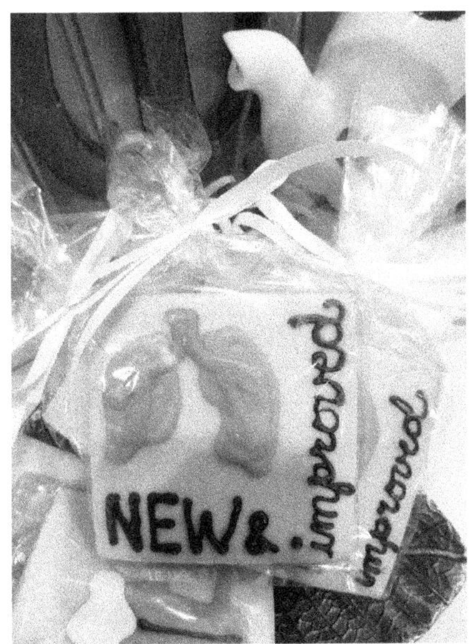

This clever lung-themed cookie bouquet
was better than a get-well card.
Thanks, A. Haut!

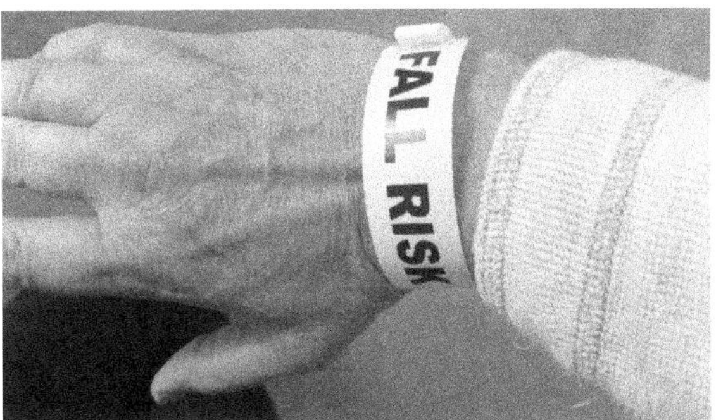

My discharge instructions included
this cautionary bracelet.

Chapter Six

Bucket List

Tim McGraw's song "Live Like You Were Dying" probably has encouraged thousands of people to develop a bucket list and made many people realize one of my favorite sayings: *No one promised you tomorrow.* The challenge for most everyone is deciding what to write down on a list in the first place, then having a goal to check them off before it is too late. Looking back, I believe most people have had bucket-list opportunities when you don't expect them. You just have to take advantage of the opportunity. That sense of urgency may happen, then work happens, life happens and, "Dang, I wish I had done that!"

My dad had a few things he wanted to do but, like many people, he worked until it was too late. He learned he had terminal liver cancer, and his priorities quickly changed. He was practicing law in his early seventies when the news came. It was a terrible way to die. I promised myself I would not allow that to happen to me. When I made that promise to myself, I had a job that required a lot of traveling. I tried to turn those travels into adventures. I am not sure if I would have bought my home in Matagorda without that promise.

During the orientation given to transplant patients, they use the words "your new normal." I hated to hear that. I wanted my old normal. People who have hobbies are told you can't do certain things or travel to certain places. Your bucket list, before you were told you had your disease or that you needed a transplant, is probably based on those hobbies. This was not easy for me to comprehend. It is not easy for anyone. We are told about many lifestyle changes, diet restrictions, and limited exposure to certain environments, crowds, or places where your compromised immunity could be fatal. It means you are somewhat tethered to your hospital for labs, med changes, and setbacks. When I travel, I always look up in advance where the nearest good hospital is located.

Some people go back to work because the high cost of the disease and now everything after the transplant, such as medication, is very expensive. Some of the people in my transplant group were able to retire or were sometimes forced to retire. You still have to manage a new lifestyle with added financial burdens that none of us never planned for. The bucket list is so important because we all need to have things to look forward to doing, planning, having fun, being challenged, learning, and enjoying life.

My bucket list still includes a fishing trip with Jim every year. We had only missed one year since our first trip to Florida in 1972 while attending the University of Kentucky. We had decided these trips were important and each trip would be an adventure.

One of our best adventures was tarpon fishing in Costa Rica, but we never had a bad trip. We learned to "half-ass" fly-fish for bonefish in the Bahamas a few times. We hired a crusty fly-fishing guide in Tampa Bay a couple of times named Captain Shirley to teach us to saltwater fly-fish. I asked him if I was ready to fish for tarpon and he said with the profanity of a crusty football coach that I might as well go bear hunting with a BB gun. I saw him in the bay a few months ago hollering at some new fly-fishermen who had hired him, and I laughed. My new lungs will not slow me down from half-ass doing anything if I can help it.

Jim and I always have a wonderful time, no matter where we fish. We've caught a variety of fish together, but the fishing has always been better than the catching. My transplant and COVID nearly messed up our string of trips, but by fifty-one weeks, our string continued on the last week of 2021 in Florida. We fished offshore Tampa Bay in Jim's boat. It was a great day.

My bucket list caused me to never miss the opportunity to go to a Jimmy Buffett concert if he was in the area. These normally included an outdoor venue preceded with thousands of "Parrot Heads" tailgating all day while consuming plenty of margaritas.

A few years back, Gale was notified that he would be performing in Houston at the Toyota Center. Tickets were available for American Express Gold Card members. We thought, "Inside concert with American Express holders and no tailgating?" But what the hell. We did not want to miss it. As we waited in line to get in, no one was wearing Hawaiian shirts (except for a very few of us), nor shark-fin hats, hula skirts, or with "cheeseburger in paradise" signs. As we entered the arena, there was a mature lady in a mink coat (I kid you not) telling us she had never been to a Jimmy Buffett concert and was looking forward to it. I told her "Ma'am, you still haven't." When it was time for "fins to the left, fins to the right," the crowd was politely sitting in their arena chairs and seemed annoyed by true Parrot Heads standing in their way and dancing. In hindsight, if that was not a bucket-list event, nothing was.

During my professional career, my goal was to make sure I did not miss opportunities related to travel requirements. I never wanted to regret not doing some of the great experiences in life these trips provided. This was more important to me than getting a promotion or a few jumps up the corporate totem pole. My various jobs had always required attending a lot of meetings and conferences. These trips always allowed for great opportunities to see new places. No organization holds a conference in shithole places.

My job in Washington, D.C., also provided many opportunities for me to experience interesting places and meet people that I would have only dreamed about while growing up in rural Kentucky.

Attending the Breeders' Cup, Kentucky Derby, World Series, and Final Four all rank as bucket-list experiences that I hope to do again.

My bucket list includes items that only a fisherman would appreciate. Every fly-fisherman has a bucket list to catch a tarpon, a permit, and a bonefish on the same day. It is called a "grand slam," and one day this will be marked off my list.

There have been trips that were not on my list but ended up being a bucket-list event. For example, I received a call from former co-worker and friend Eric Maidla. I helped him get his new technology company started as a spin-out from Noble Corp. Out of the blue, he called me and wanted to know if Gale and I would like to take a trip to fish for peacock bass in the Brazilian Amazon.

He and his wife, Lydia, were from Brazil, and he had always wanted to see the Amazon Rainforest. He moved to the U.S. to attend Louisiana State University, but they still had family in Brazil.

Eric said we would be accompanied by his two sons and family from Brazil, as well as a couple of business colleagues from Norway. Being from Brazil, they helped us overcome any language barriers pretty easily. It was short notice, but since we would only need to cover our flight to Manaus, a city on the forks of the Amazon and Negro rivers, the decision was a no-brainer.

We toured the area where the rivers met, and then we flew to Barcelos, a small river town. We stayed on a houseboat that cruised up the Rio Negro, where we ate great food and had plenty of Caipirinhas cocktails at the end of each successful day of fishing and sightseeing. We each had small fishing boats and very good guides. This was a once-in-a-lifetime experience, and the great fishing was just a bonus.

No one ever knows when their life will be put on hold. Many of my travels were because I had learned from how my dad put things off until it was too late. This caused me to reprioritize. I now have a second chance, and Gale and I are working on our updated list.

My Matagorda friend John Crenshaw invited me on a fishing trip to Panama, which has great tuna fishing that's advertised as thirty miles from nowhere. I told John that my new life required me to be thirty miles from somewhere, just in case. It is a compromise worth the risk.

My last bucket list item includes making it to heaven. I hope it is a while before I do that last one!

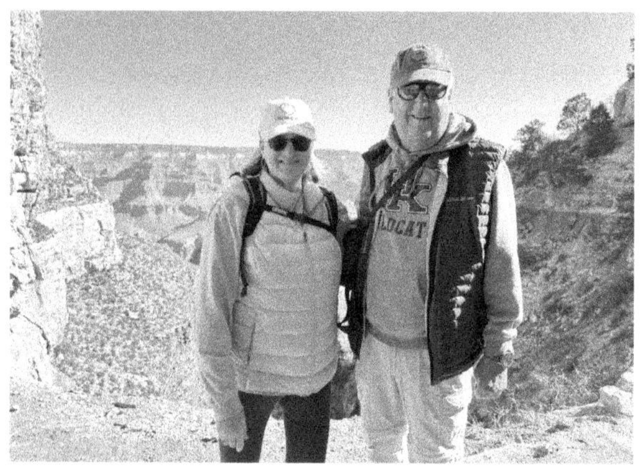

Another adventure:
Hiking the Grand Canyon— Year Two.

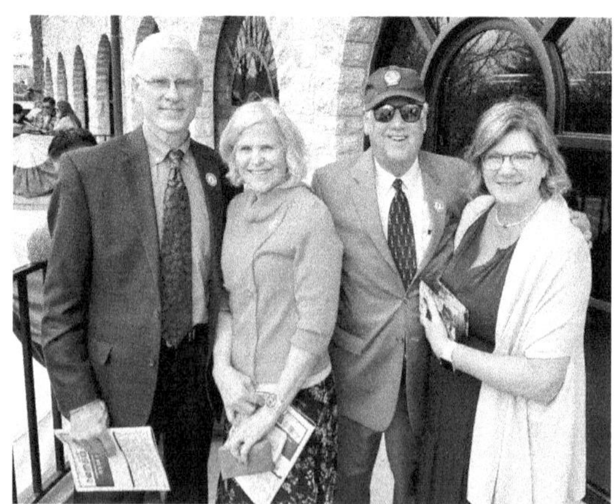

Having the best day at Breeders' Cup at Keeneland
in Kentucky with Sue, David, and Gale.

Chapter Seven

The Letters

May 2021

The month after I returned from the hospital, I re-read all the notes and get-well cards I received. There were a lot from all over the country. I decided to have thank-you cards printed to send out as soon as possible. It started with a Robert Earl Keen quote: "It feels so good to be feelin' good again." The note continued: "We are grateful for our good doctors, our many friends and family. Your prayers and support have been a tremendous help and we are eternally thankful. This will be a long and challenging recovery, but knowing the worst is behind us, and with all of the support we have received, we are confident the future is bright. Gale and I hope we can one day thank you in person."

I still have the list, and we intend to do just that.

I recently learned that my primary transplant doctor was leaving the University of Kentucky and moving to Houston.

I hated the news and wrote this letter:

Dear Dr. Baz:

Gale and I wanted to make sure we expressed our appreciation for what you have done for us before you left Lexington. Your expertise and compassion saved my life—so how can we ever express that gratitude in words? We wish you all the best in your new challenge and know a lot of lives will be saved because of you.

We lived in Houston for a number of years before we moved to Kentucky. Houston is a wonderful, diverse, and opportunistic place to live. We lived near Memorial Park, which you will find is a haven within such a large city. We also owned a weekend home in Matagorda; a wonderful getaway place that molded our lives and brought joy to our souls.

You will always be in our hearts (and my lungs) as we know what you have done will provide us with many years of happiness that we would not have otherwise experienced.

With much love and respect,

Tom Williams

The thank-you-for-my-lungs letter

There are strict rules on the process to contact an organ donor family. You can't use your last name or address; it is required to send it through the system that procures organs (the United Network for Organ Sharing). If the family wishes to respond, then there is a system for that, too.

All transplant recipients I have met are so grateful for this gift and find it difficult that there is no one they can directly thank. It took me a while to figure out what I wanted to say, and I added that letter below. After five months, I have not yet heard back. In speaking to others who have received a transplant, fewer than half ever hear back. No one knows the circumstances, only that this generous gift saved my life.

April 9, 2021

To my lung donor family:

My name is Tom, I am 68 and I live in Kentucky with my wife, Gale, and our dog, Colonel. This past week I passed my ninety-day anniversary receiving two lungs because of your family's generosity. I am alive, I am feeling good and healthy today, thanks to you.

In early 2018 I was a busy guy living in Houston, working as president of a not-for-profit oil-and-gas research organization. I developed a cough and shortness of breath, and my wife convinced me to visit our family doctor. It was not long before I was diagnosed with a lung disease called Idiopathic Pulmonary Fibrosis (IPF). I learned it was a progressive disease with no cure. The disease made it prohibitive for me to continue my job, which required extensive travel. It became increasingly evident that my only shot at life was a lung transplant.

After a lot of research, thought, and prayer, we moved back home from Texas to Kentucky near our family and our medical center. There I participated in pulmonary rehab and met some incredible doctors. I was evaluated for a transplant and, eventually in the spring of 2020 in the midst of COVID, was put on the list. I had to have oxygen most of the time and waited thirty weeks for a match. We had a couple of dry runs and then I received a call from my doctor incredibly early one morning. The next day, January 6, a miracle happened to me following what must have been a tragic event for you. I think about this often with some conflict of guilt and gratitude.

This experience obviously has changed my life in many ways, as I have a greater appreciation for life (and not just mine), a deeper love and gratitude for my wife, a greater appreciation for my closest friends, and understanding how the power of prayer from an amazing network of friends, family, and acquaintances across the country truly works.

I have never been a patient person, so naturally I have a feeling of urgency to get on with my life, travel, to be productive again, and so I am working hard to build myself up physically. I also know my road to recovery is still long and does not lend itself to my impatience. Through this, I have also developed tremendous gratitude for this gift, thanks to you. I would like to thank you on the phone, in person, or whatever you choose. I mainly wanted you to know the impact you have made with your gift of life to me and my family.

God Bless and thank you,

Tom

No response yet. Some in our support group have written similar letters, and several have had a response from the family. Every circumstance is different. As recipients, we are grateful and guilty at the same time. We all hope the family knows we have been blessed by their generosity.

Chapter Eight

A Year to Wait—A Year to Recover

Tarpon fishing can be hours of boredom followed by moments of total pandemonium. Many fishermen like me live for this thrill, which requires a lot of patience, skill, and strength to successfully hook up and land one of the best fighting fish that swims.

This is not unlike the proper mental and physical preparation needed to meet many of the unexpected challenges that life throws one's way. Tarpon fishing is different from most other pursuits in that you can fish all day, only get a few strikes, a couple of good jumps before the fish throws the hook, then it gets off and you still end up having a pretty good day. The tarpon was going back anyway. How many times can we claim success and not even land the fish we have pursued for hours?

When I was diagnosed with my lung disease in March 2018, I started keeping detailed health records in my business journal, which I had used for years. If I could record health factors that documented changes one way or the other, it would help me going forward and hopefully help my doctors. In documenting all of this, my days of feeling decent vs. feeling lousy were recorded: my vitals, oxygen level, weather, any exercise I did, what meds I took, how I was doing and, fortunately, a few entries of "pretty good day today." In doing this, it also helped in communicating with my doctors and probably helped me get on the transplant list sooner than later. It demonstrated that I would keep up with my medications and lower my risk of rejection.

In business I learned to document my activities for the day, record my objectives for the next day and week, and review them before I went home. So, by the end of the week, I could see what I accomplished and could then add new objectives and goals instead of making a list of catch-up items. I recorded conversations that I could go back and review. Applying this to my health, the objective was to do what I needed in order to first get on and then to stay on the transplant list. I *had* to record my vitals; I *needed* to exercise, even when I felt tired or bad; I *had* to force myself to eat, even though my appetite was gone; I *had* to read and research something/anything to keep my mind going. This was all pretty abstract stuff compared to running an organization, creating business development activities, and then keeping a professional network growing, but it was a tremendous help. Documenting demonstrates accountability.

Upon my diagnosis, I knew I would not "hook up" with any tarpon in the near term, and really there was no way to prepare myself for the emotional changes I was about to take on. All of this is compounded by seeing similar frustrations that Gale had to deal with. I knew she was going through an emotional roller coaster in dealing with these life changes. We both knew we were going to get through this. We knew we were blessed with family and friends to help. The disease and the waiting were more difficult than we had anticipated.

It helped us that we were blessed with our dog, Colonel, who provided a tremendous amount of emotional support and joy. We also had a rescue dog, Rascal, who was one of those "I am lucky and happy to be here" creatures. He did not make it to the end of our transplant journey, but if there was ever anything that showed us how to survive and be happy about life, it was him.

I did not record all my disappointments and frustrations in my journal (as I probably should have). What does one say or write down when they just had a really bad day or, worse, lost a friend or family member and can't go to the funeral? Then there's the letdown of a dry run, and the withdrawals of not being able to do the things you worked hard for and now were not able to do. Funny enough, all UK football and basketball scores (and comments) are in the journal.

It was not easy to go back and read my daily journal entries. When the evaluation process started, my doctors were monitoring my health. I provided them with additional data. They knew I would not get on the official waiting list until my condition deteriorated enough to warrant the transplant vs. others more deserving.

In January 2020, they decided it was time for me to go through the evaluation and eliminate any issues that would prohibit or complicate the transplant. Mine was a three-day evaluation scheduled for Jan. 21, so naturally I went fishing in Florida, then we returned on the Sunday before my tests.

They poked and prodded every place on my body. On the third day, they did a heart catheterization, where they found a blockage and had to put in a stent. They told me I was very lucky that they found it, and it was successful. I could have had a heart attack and died.

I would need to start taking a statin and other meds, so I would not be eligible to get on the list for a few months. Bad news sort of rolled off our backs by that time anyway.

My UK physical therapist, Megan, helped me get into transplant shape and especially get back in shape after the transplant. She was the inspiration I needed, learning how to manage my competitive nature. I always did more than the goal she set for me that day. I also needed to get several vaccinations and some dental work out of the way, which would be more effective before the transplant.

The stent never improved my health or energy level. I was on oxygen most of the time to keep my levels in the 90s.

The cardiologists monitored my condition and added Plavix to my daily medications on Feb. 4. I would continue Esbriet, which meant all the bad side effects would not go away. My coughing became worse, even though it was bad before, which meant less sleep and more headaches, but I kept working out and trying to keep myself ready. I was able to plumb an oxygen line into our bedroom so the loud vibration of the machine would not keep us awake. I also had a smaller portable oxygen machine so I could travel around town and use it while I worked out and walked.

I spoke to my friend Bobby Dolence from time to time, and he kept my spirits up and provided support. He provided me with a lot of information about how to prepare for a post-transplant life, as well as plenty of data to read and questions to ask my doctors.

Our wedding anniversary is the first Saturday in April. I have a difficult time remembering dates and convinced Gale I would always remember the first Saturday in April because it is a month before the Derby. No true Kentuckian would ever forget that date, the first Saturday in May. It was also the weekend of the Final Four basketball tournament, which is a time every Kentucky Wildcat looks forward to but is usually disappointed. This being my wedding anniversary, I figured I would always be happy, even if UK lost. Such was the case on April 4, 2020, when we celebrated at home with a great steak, a good bottle of wine, and perfect weather. There would be no UK in the Final Four, but there was always next year. It was one of the few days when I did not have a headache, and my coughing was not too bad.

COVID was starting to become a major concern. There were no rules or analog guidelines. The government was making stuff up as this progressed. We figured this was especially bad for us. I was instructed to avoid crowds as much as possible.

April is also Keeneland racing time, but COVID and new guidelines caused the event to postpone. I would have missed it anyway, and we would have to wait another year or two. I made a note in the journal that I felt confined, like four walls and no jukebox. I also had several entries of severe cough, fatigue, and headache. My UK doctors decided to do another heart catheterization on April 29 because I was feeling pretty bad. The report came back good. They started me on Prednisone, and I immediately knew I would feel much worse with less rest. I was correct, and the cough did not subside. The steroids are a necessary evil.

At this point, most of my days were filled with reading, followed by an hour or so workout (a walk) while Gale worked from home. I was cooking a lot more than normal, which was not easy with no appetite.

The date my mom died was May 15, which was the day before my dad's birthdate. The only way I recall these important days is because of Outlook reminders and my sister Sue, who is good at reminding me of the dates I need to remember. I then record them in my diary. Had Gale known this, I may have been forced to have a real date for our anniversary. Sue and I agreed to travel to our hometown of Campbellsville the next year to honor what would have been our dad's 100th birthday. (We actually made it to the cemetery seventy-five miles away, although I had my doubts at the time.) It was a good day.

On June 6, I went to the UK clinic for labs and various tests. I was told I was going on the list! I could stop taking Plavix, so I would start feeling a little better. To celebrate, Gale had her sister Holly give me my first haircut in about four months. I think she did not want me to get the call and then look like a bum when we arrived at the hospital. We packed a "go" bag and made a plan.

Then the long wait began.

I was wrong about feeling a little better, because many of my journal entries reminded me how I was becoming weaker, with bad headaches, fatigue, and joint and muscle pain. It was also difficult to keep my oxygen level up, especially when I exercised. I was given certain exercises to help with my recovery. The commitment to do them every day ended up being a blessing.

Getting calls and cards from many of my old friends and former co-workers was a tremendous emotional lift. I made a note in my journal of every call, email, and letter I received that summer and fall.

I was also wrapping up some commitments with my past work, including the Interstate Oil and Gas Commission. It was a wonderful diversion and made me feel like I could still contribute to something worthwhile. I had "conned" one of my best friends, Lanny Schoeling, into taking over my committee work, which was a big relief, and he would do a better job than me anyway. We have continued to speak by phone almost every week or so.

Dr. Baz called at 4:30 a.m. on July 18 for what would be our first dry run. They called us right when we were arriving at the hospital to let us know the lungs were not suitable. It was a short and sad ride back home. The next week, I was evaluated and assured that something would happen before long. It was good to have that behind us.

My coordinating nurse, Ashley, was a huge help during this process. She was my communication link to UK. We spoke at least once or twice a week, and she will be a buddy for life.

UK added additional medication to alleviate my pain and discomfort. They all have side effects, it seems. My headaches were frequent and got worse, and my blood pressure was low, usually around 88/60 most of the time. It became difficult to keep my oxygen level up while trying to stay semi-active, so we had to get a more powerful oxygen machine.

The Kentucky Derby was now set for September because of the COVID delay. My internal schedule was a mess. No lungs yet, so I figured I'd live to see at least one more derby. My dogs, Colonel and Rascal, and I watched the races on TV and bet on the horses all day online. I had gone to Spaulding's Bakery, and we shared a dozen doughnuts. Colonel watched the races with me between naps, and Rascal was interested in the next doughnut. I lost a little money. I told Gale that Colonel provided bad advice, but we both had a good day. It was a nice diversion.

COVID was taking its toll on the country, but we were isolated anyway. I realized how lucky we both were because we were able to get along so well. You never know about things when you are secluded. It became clear that Gale got along better with our dogs than me, but still being in the top three was not all that bad. Both our birthdays were in September, and we had several phone calls with many old friends.

I limited watching the national news. It was all bad and, after thirty minutes, I usually had my fill. The election rhetoric on TV just made it worse.

Low energy, cough, and headaches continued to get a little worse throughout October and November. It seemed like we would never get the call. Gale cooked a lot of food for Thanksgiving because she was intent on celebrating. It was a grand meal. A lot of leftovers. We spent most such holidays with the Toombs, but not this year. It was difficult to not think about fishing, being on the water, and playing card games with our friends. This was what I always enjoyed the most about Thanksgiving week.

On Dec. 8, Dr. Baz called and said there was a possible donor. We checked in and waited. We were given COVID tests and Gale was allowed to stay with me. Her sister Holly was on the road from her home in London, Kentucky, which is seventy-five miles south of Lexington, to help take care of the dogs.

After twenty-four hours in the hospital, the trip resulted in a dry run. The lungs were not viable for transplant. We learned during my pre-op that my chest had shrunk because my lungs were now smaller, and they needed to look for a smaller donor. At six feet and normal build, I thought a five-foot-nine-or-ten-inch person may be easier to find anyway. We came home and I fixed an Eagle Rare Manhattan. It was my first bourbon in months. It was not the best day, but the bourbon helped.

Two days later, we made the hard decision that it would be Rascal's last day. He had a very rough six weeks, and the vet said his time was over. It was a very sad time for us.

We decorated for a low-key Christmas. All that I wanted was new lungs, but it looked like it might not happen until after the holidays. We enjoyed the holidays the best we could. We discouraged family visits—Adam, his wife, Liz, and our granddaughter, Olive, plus Gale's family—because we could not afford to get a cold, or worse, COVID.

On Jan. 1, 2021, I made a note in my journal that it was week thirty on the waiting list, and the waiting was hard. We got the news that my sister Sue and brother-in-law David had COVID. Gale's sister Holly and my sister Sue were our safety nets.

On Jan. 5 at 4:45 a.m., we received a call from Dr. Baz. He said they had some lungs and they seemed to be a good match. COVID highly complicated the process, and we understood the challenges. Having gone through dry runs before, we were excited, yet it was tempered.

I was assigned a room via phone, and we went straight there, where they did blood work and we waited. Early the next morning, on Jan. 6, I was headed to surgery. I was too numb to think about the enormity of the moment, but I knew I was ready for whatever happened next. We had no idea what was going on in the rest of the world that day, and we could care less. To us, Jan. 6 will always be Transplant Day. Our friends also reminded us later it was also the day of the Epiphany.

Gale took over the diary duties, and her notes were extremely important and much easier to read than mine. She also set up a network of everyone who had supported us. It was a pretty amazing process. There were prayer and support groups that were set up to initially contact my sisters Sue and Janie or my friends Rich or Lanny, and then they would contact others. I have no idea how many people were rooting for us, but we received a lot of cards, even from some people I hardly knew, like a Sunday school class from my hometown. This all was amazing and humbling to us.

Gale noted surgery began at 6 a.m. by Dr. K. The OR nurse gave her updates every two hours. At 5 p.m., Gale was told the surgery was over. Dr. K told her at 5:30 that it was successful.

What a stressful day that must have been for her. There were some challenges but no major complications. Dr. Baz told her to get some rest until tomorrow.

The next day I was on a ventilator and sedated when Dr. Baz told Gale it was evident the lungs had developed pneumonia. They were treating it with heavy doses of antibiotics and prednisone. I would be on the ventilator for a few more days. Gale watched the screen as the bronchial scope was inserted into the new lungs. Gale wrote how she observed the removal of the scope, which was evidently painful considering my strong reaction. They gave me morphine and a muscle paralytic. Although I was heavily sedated, I recalled sounds, pain, Gale's presence, and Dr. Baz's urgency. He stayed and monitored my condition for a long time.

Gale said that Ashley showed up to check on me and delivered my new hat from the UK transplant with "#437" of lung transplants embroidered on the side. I have worn the cap many times since.

COVID protocols were being made up as they went. There was no analog, so mistakes were bound to be made. One of the dumber rules was to send Gale home for the night, so it was completely possible that she could catch COVID before she was allowed to visit the next morning.

The next day, Gale wrote about how I had a bad night, had developed delirium, and they had to increase the sedation. The nurse said that this was my response to fighting the infection. I must have been fighting like hell that night and day. I finally became alert enough to recognize my surroundings, open my eyes, and squeeze Gale's hand.

While I became aware of where I was, I was still heavily sedated to tolerate the pain. My first lucid thought was, "Oh, crap. I have an unopened bottle of Blanton's at home." Perhaps not so lucid after all! When I was heavily sedated and in pain, I would wake to Gale playing music like Kenny Chesney's "Boats," with lyrics / Boats / Vessels of freedom / Harbors of healing /, and I was immediately in a better frame of mind.

Gale made several notes about my frustration at the inability to communicate.

On the 10th, they learned I had an infection and had to maintain antibiotics. Dr. K. wanted to get me off sedation to check my response, and Gale said it appeared I was alert for an hour, even when on the ventilator. He said he wanted to get me off the ventilator as soon as possible. It was Dr. Baz's call. They thought it was good news, but I had a fever and they put me back on sedation so I could rest.

I would sometimes think I was on the Gulf in my boat, the water was gin clear, the wind was calm, and I could see birds working ahead of me. Many times, my ICU nurse would remind me that it was time for my pills, then reality would quickly set in.

The next couple of days were slow progress, fighting off the infection, while the physical therapists were doing what they could to get me moving. They told Gale I was in good shape and had a strong will to move.

On the 13th, they found a third bacterial infection, but Dr. Baz said the antibiotics were working. They lowered the sedation drugs, and I was more alert. Gale played music throughout this time, and she wrote that I was happy when she played Jack Johnson. Happy music like Kenny Chesney, Jack Johnson, Jimmy Buffett, and others was a tremendous help while I was confined.

The next day, they confirmed I was in rejection. The decision was to up the prednisone dose to 1,000 mg for three days. They later did another bronchoscopy, which confirmed the medications meant to fight the rejection were working. I sometimes recall the pain to this day and wake up with cold sweats.

Gale wrote that it was frustrating for me to not be able to communicate, and I was in a lot of discomfort. Dr. Baz discussed my situation out of the room to let Gale know how serious things were. She had full confidence that he was being aggressive to save my life while also realizing the toll this was having on my system.

I recall one moment when I was on a high dosage and they were working on me in my ICU room. Gale said my blood pressure and vitals were rapidly spiking and then dropping. I felt like I was in a dark place, in a lot of pain, and that I might not make it. It was the only time I felt like I was ready for whatever happened, as long as the pain would end. It was like, "Please, God, I need some relief." The next thing I remember was Gale's voice, then I figured everything was okay. She probably had a Jack Johnson song on to take my mind away from what I was going through.

They removed the ventilator on Saturday the 16th, and I will never forget that first breath for the rest of my life. It seemed like an eternity before I could breathe on my own, but it felt strange that my normal breathing seemed abnormal. Gale said I could whisper and was alert.

The physical therapists were very helpful and encouraging from that point on.

Things did not progress on a steady path, however, because I experienced delirium. As I recall, I had some very wild, crazy thoughts going through my mind. Looking at the notes, it is somewhat embarrassing to read some of the things I was thinking, especially as Gale wrote that I told her that one of the get-well cards she showed me was from U.S. Secretary of Transportation Pete Buttigieg. Where the hell did that thought come from? Gale corrected me the next day, and I told her I knew it, that it was actually from his husband. How crazy is that! My friend Kelly sent several cards, all funny and all very much needed.

My ICU nurses were amazing as they helped me through this exceedingly difficult time. I can't say enough good things about their compassion and hard work. I must have been a handful with delirium and my inability to properly communicate. We wrote down everyone's name and did our best to thank them (and apologize) after the ordeal.

I was finally able to eat real food (so to speak) on the 19th, although Gale had to make a run to the cafeteria for some hot sauce to make it tolerable. I considered Jell-O shots made with Tabasco at one point. This was a good sign that I was getting back. She brought me a supply of snacks so I could eat something before they made me take pills every three hours. Otherwise, they would mess with my stomach. I was not a fan of the hospital food, either.

Over the next couple of days, I was able to read, speak on the phone, and do some exercises on my own, but I was still on oxygen. I recall a get-well video from our granddaughter, Olive, that perked me up.

The music that Gale played for me was very helpful, and I was finally able to get some rest without sedation. On the 22nd, they moved me out of ICU to the other side of the same floor, and I walked from one side of the hospital floor to the other. This was good exercise and allowed me to check in on my ICU nurses. At that time, they said I would be able to go home in three to four days. The UK physical therapists were a tremendous help.

They monitored my blood and vitals continuously. I was alert enough to watch UK basketball games on TV, but the team sucked in 2021. The national news was intolerable during this time, so I did not try to keep up. I did some reading, but my comprehension was low. Fishing magazines were about as deep of reading as I could manage.

I took over my diary duties on the 23rd, which was a big mistake! From this part on, the delirium, shaky hands, and a fuzzy mind took too much control over my cognitive writing and thinking ability.

Daily X-rays at 5 a.m. and regular nebulizer treatments got my days started with me in a bad mood. The hospital beds were designed for short people, and I recall raising hell every time I was moved from room to room until I got a bed extension.

I was sent back to ICU on the 25th because of dehydration. At least Gale was able to wrestle the journal away from me to document what was taking place for a couple of days.

While in the ICU, I did my best to get my mind to take me to my "happy place" to escape the intense condition. My thoughts went something like: *I made the last turn and headed across the bridge. I rolled down the window on my truck to breathe the salty air, turning on the stereo to hear Leon Russell sing "Back to the Island." Colonel had patiently slept in the passenger seat during the two-hour trip, and then he sprung to life, jumped across the console and into my lap. He wanted to share his joy of being in Matagorda and get his fill of the salty air. It was time to pop the top on the beer that had been chilling on the drive down from Houston. The bay was calm and the fishing would be good. I dared not look in the rearview mirror because everything good was in front of me and not behind. The next thing I recall was, "Mr. Williams, it is 5 a.m. and time for your morning X-ray."* The reality of that moment did not spoil the joy of my memory. I swear I could smell the salty air.

I laugh today when I hear John Prine's funny song "Other Side of Town" where he describes how his mind took him away from his current unhappy situation. I can always relate to this.

One of the requirements for discharge is passing the "swallow test." I was telling the technician they should give the *Cool Hand Luke* test, and I bet her I could swallow fifty boiled eggs like Paul Newman did in the movie. She really had no idea what I was talking about, because *Cool Hand Luke* was made in the '60s before her time. She must have thought I was still delirious. I finally passed the test on the 26th and got the okay from the physical therapist. We were sure I would be able to immediately go home.

The hospital provided us with a discharge list. That's when it really struck us that there was so much work for Gale to do at home: managing my forty pills a day and taking my vitals, which needed to be regularly monitored and recorded. The medications caused my sugar levels to jump, so I had to do blood tests and get insulin shots. I also had blood-thinner shots. I hated pricking my finger twice a day. Thank goodness we had help.

Jim's wife, Cindy, arrived from Florida ready to help us before I arrived home. My last test was another bronc and, sure enough, Dr. Baz said they found some rejection. Crap! I was sent back to ICU for an infusion. The additional medications were not good on my system, and I was feeling pretty bad. I also had significant back pain from the uncomfortable beds. Additional pain medication was needed. Physical therapy was very helpful to get me through this. My IV meds were through a PICC line, and X-rays and nebulizer treatments continued.

On Groundhog Day, Cindy's daughter Heather had another boy, whom I thought should be named Phil in honor of the Punxsutawney groundhog. I was overruled. We told her to go be with Heather in Tampa. We had no idea when I would be discharged to go home, but she said she was not going to leave.

The next day I celebrated by walking the halls with no walker. I was more than ready to go home. We went over food and medications with the pharmacist to prepare us. Gale brought me a breakfast roll from DV8, one of our favorite bakeries, which made my levels jump exceedingly high. So, they gave me a double dose of insulin. It was worth it. I asked her to bring me a poster and some markers to make a sign saying, "Free Tom." I planned to put it on my window because I believed it was my best chance to get out.

My surgeon, Dr. K, checked in on me most days and would let me in on information from my chart that he thought I may not have been told and needed to know. During this time, I had grown a full gray beard, and my hair had grown longer than normal. He offered to bring me a razor and find a nurse to clean me up. It became a running joke between us as I told him I was going to look like an old hippie until I was discharged. The guy really lifted my spirits during this long stay.

One of the transplant doctors was Dr. Michael Anstead, who filled in for Dr. Baz when he was on leave. He saw me over the weekend. Gale was not at the hospital when we had a serious talk. He said I was looking good but discussed how serious things had gone after the transplant. He said my preparation paid off, but that I was lucky. I learned he was an avid bike rider and he encouraged me to get on the bike trail when the weather allowed. It was good advice, and we had plenty of things to talk about on follow-up visits.

Super Bowl Sunday was Feb. 7. Hospital food service brought me a pizza to eat while watching Tampa win the game. Jim and his son Ryan were big fans and watched the game from Florida as we all spoke that day, and they were excited. Gale and Cindy were at our home. Some of the nurses who had taken care of me in the ICU stopped by my room to keep me company. They said I would be going home soon. I was discharged on the 8th. It was great to go home, and I had a good night's sleep.

Starting the next day, I was required to go to regular appointments at the transplant clinic. Fortunately, the clinic is less than two miles from our home, which was a blessing. Many transplant patients either have to spend the transition time in a hotel, with friends, or drive a long distance. Over the next year, I made many trips to the clinic weekly, then monthly. I have almost become numb to having my blood drawn. The technicians who administer the tests, like Larry and Christina, have become friends.

The first year I had some health challenges and made a few return trips to the hospital for pneumonia and aspergillus. The added medications and high levels of steroids, in addition to all my anti-rejection meds, complicated the way I felt. I ended up with sepsis after one bronc, which put me back in the hospital for a while. Reactions to the medications seemed to make me feel worse, but my doctors did their best to mitigate these problems.

I recorded everything in my journal and made sure the data were on my medical records. Before one procedure, as they thoroughly went through all my records, I told them to put brussel sprouts and broccoli on the list was well. The nurse wrote them down, but Gale was in the room and busted me when they were going over my charts before a bronc. It was worth a shot.

It was hard to gauge my progress day to day because they were bad and good, but when I looked at my diary for the year, it showed progress. One of the best things about writing all this down was to document progress. It was a long year to wait and a long year to recover. The broncs and ICU visits were bad, and so was the fatigue. At the end of Year One, I knew better days were coming.

Eventually I think all patients like me finally get to understand the medications, how your body reacts, the importance of exercise, and appreciation for all the people in the system who are dedicated to helping.

You also learn to appreciate those who helped you get through this. When we really needed help, they were there. We didn't have to ask, and we are forever grateful. This especially includes the wonderful and caring nurses I had at UK.

We were lucky because Cindy was there to help us out at home. The meds caused my blood sugar to spike, and those blood tests and shots are intimidating to anyone, unless you have the background. To this day, I do not know how to properly thank her. But this is what real friends do.

We were lucky that our family was nearby, and they were immensely helpful despite needing to balance the fear of COVID or other illnesses that would be devastating to my health. My nephew Stan, a like-minded spirit and fisherman, regularly checked in on me by phone. He always had a good story, and those calls always made my day. His weekly calls continue to brighten my spirits.

UK has a support group of pre- and post-lung transplant patients. I also found others through the Pulmonary Fibrosis Foundation, and they meet online monthly. I did not take advantage of these before my transplant, but with all the COVID restrictions and the go-to meeting apps, I was able to do so afterward.

I was determined to pass along helpful things "I wish I had known" to those who were on the waiting list. UK has a lung transplant Facebook group where issues can be passed along. Before COVID, my pulmonary rehab class provided me with a network of heart and lung patients who from time to time discussed their experiences during and after workouts. This was helpful in preparing for my recovery year.

Gale and I documented our hospital journey and prepared a list of things to help others who are now in our situation, from a patient and caregiver's perspective. We sent our list to the hospital social worker, and she circulated it to the support group for their ideas and later provided a help list to new patients. The inability to communicate was one of the most challenging things for me, but we came up with ways of improvement.

It took a few months before I could drive and get to the clinic on my own. We sometimes meet people in the transplant clinic who are much worse off than us, and this is humbling.

COVID complicated everyone's life, in particular those of us who are immunocompromised, such as transplant recipients. We must avoid catching something that would compromise our ability to survive. Unfortunately, some of the transplant patients who caught COVID did not make it. No one knows the effectiveness of the vaccines on transplant patients with no immunity, but it is crazy not to take all the precautions we can.

I had additional blood work done in addition to my normal monthly checkup, which monitors how my anti-rejection meds are doing and the toll they are taking on my other organs. Mineral deficiencies can then be dealt with. One thing they found was that my vitamin D was extremely low. I attributed this to IFS, which is short for Insufficient Fishing Syndrome. There is only one cure.

The anti-rejection medication warnings all say to avoid the sun because of the increased risk of skin cancer. But I did not get these lungs to stay inside, so I will take precautions. My long-sleeve fishing shirts, hats, buffs, and good sunscreen are packed, so I am ready to go. They also work well on my regular bike rides to the Kentucky Horse Park on the Legacy Trail.

Society and businesses have adapted to COVID by offering never-before-done services. We are taking advantage of having our supplies, groceries, and food delivered. We would have never dreamed of this as possible a few years ago. Just looking back on the short time period from 2020 to 2022, it is remarkable how things have changed.

Lab results indicate the toll that the medications are having on my other organs, bones, and energy level. I was told about the trade-offs, but it still pisses me off. No matter how hard I work to mitigate these problems, there are going to be problems.

Year Two of recovery, despite COVID barriers, was much better than Year One. That first year was not smooth sailing. Even though I was able to get out most every day to walk or ride my new e-bike and do some limited fishing and traveling, there have been plenty of challenges. I knew there would be a good deal of bumps in the road, but they were difficult to accept at the time. I realize I must continue to fight hard in order for things to eventually get better. I have a big tarpon to catch.

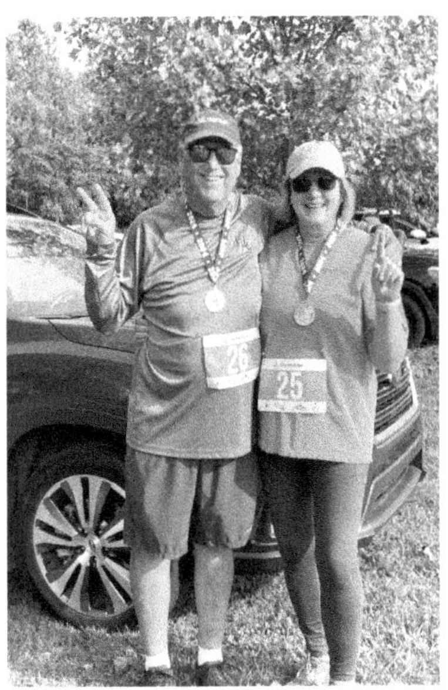

Taking on a 5K challenge in 2024.

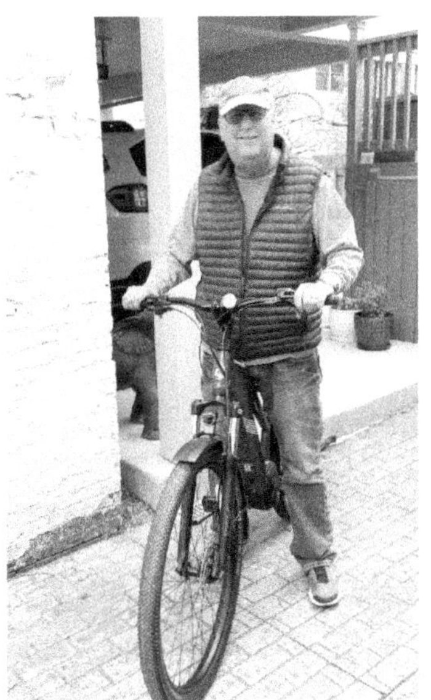

New e-bike after transplant.
The best investment!
April 2021

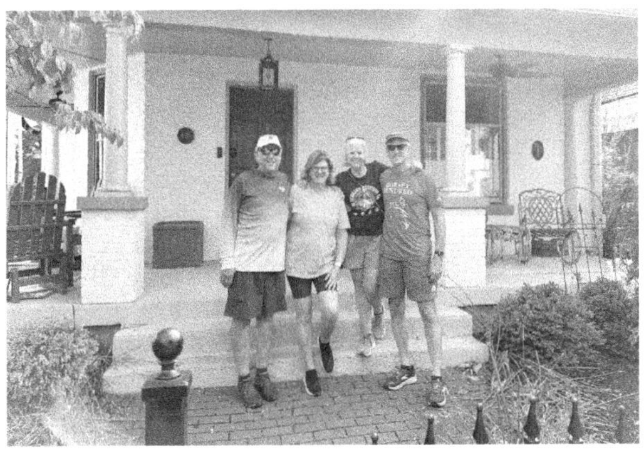

First three-mile charity walk after transplant with
Sue (my sister) and David Shaw.

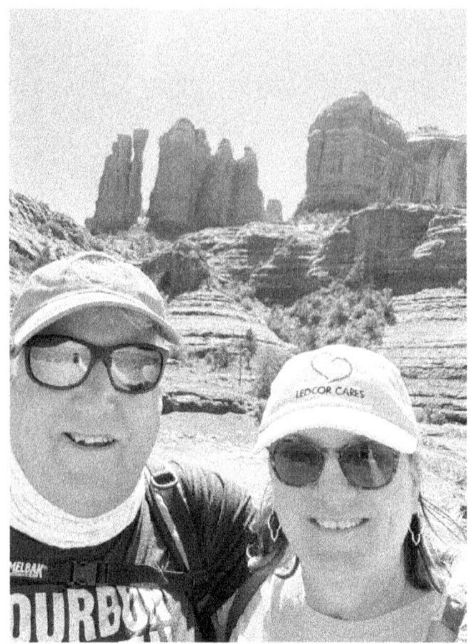

Seeing the sights with a hike in
Sedona, Arizona—Year Two.

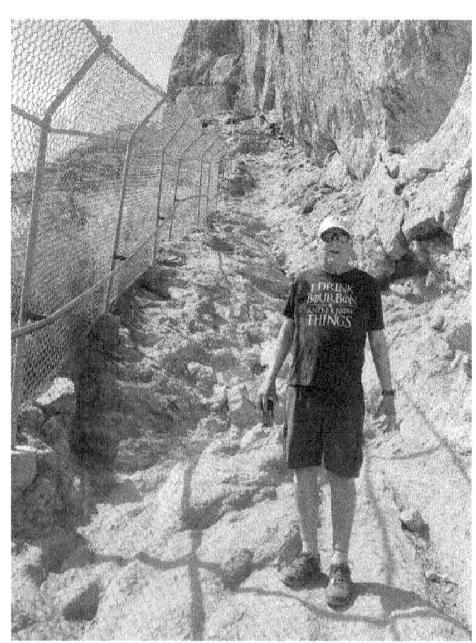

Climbing Camelback Mountain while
overweight and out of shape—Year Two.

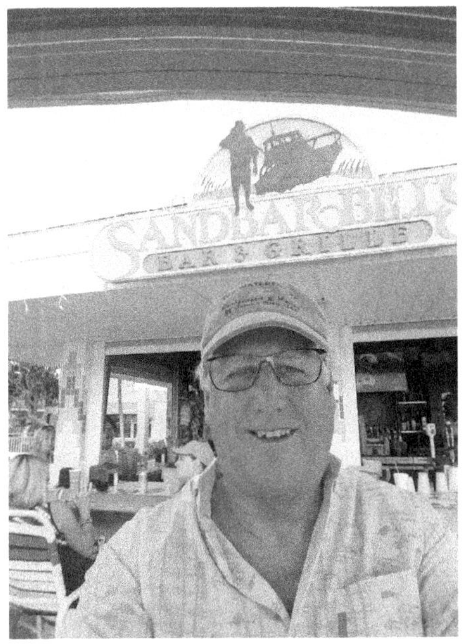

Enjoying every moment at
my happy place: St. Pete Beach, Florida.

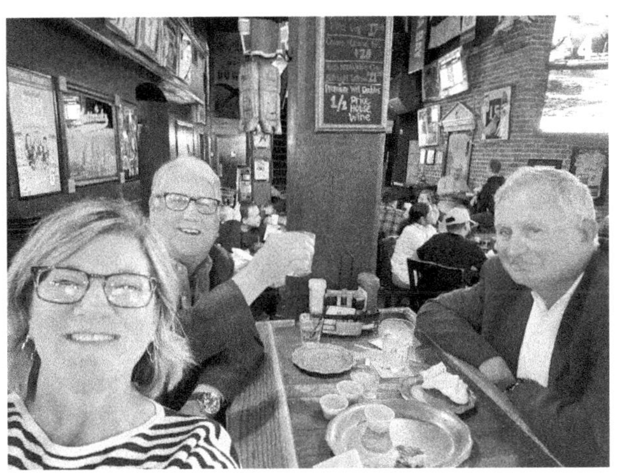

Celebrating my first transplant anniversary
in Tampa, Florida, with Jim Toombs and Gale.
Jan. 6, 2022

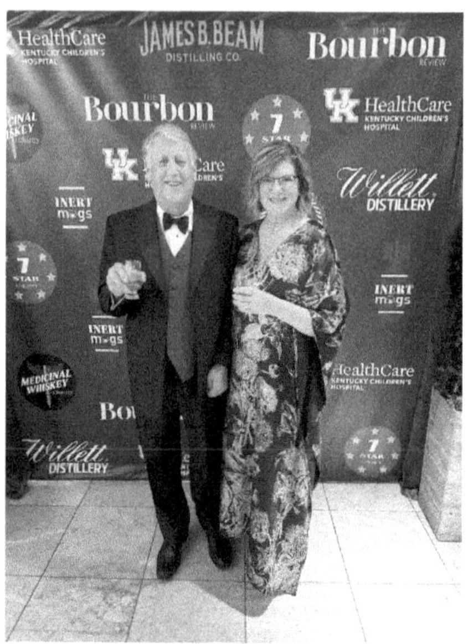

A toast at the 2023 Medicinal Whiskey Winter Gala, which benefits Kentucky Children's Hospital and the UK Transplant Center.

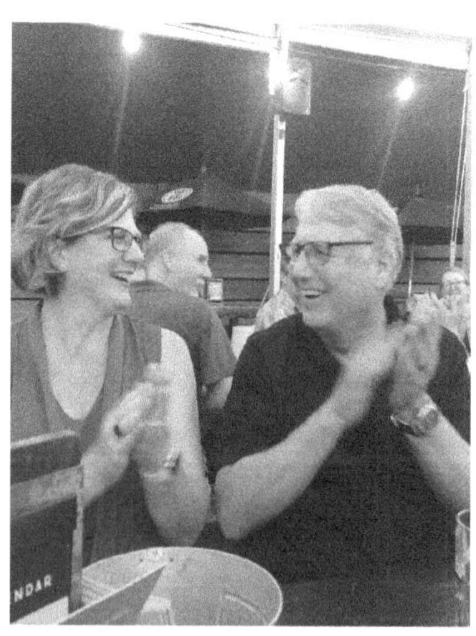

We made it!
Kicking off Year Three.

Epilogue

It took about a year after my best friend Jim's death to get back to finishing this book. Gale and I made the trip to Florida to celebrate my three-year lung anniversary on my transplant date Jan. 6. But when the day came, I did not feel like celebrating. I felt guilty.

There was comfort in being at his home to toast a life well-lived and to thank Gale and Cindy for helping me make this milestone, as we had done for the past two years.

Jim had a heart attack and died unexpectedly in Kentucky in February 2023 while attending a relative's funeral. He and Cindy did not stay with us on that trip because Gale and I had planned to be out of town to see my nephew, Stan. Somehow that week we both caught COVID. We had just been at their home in Florida a couple of weeks prior and celebrated my two-year lung anniversary together. We were lucky we had the vaccine and medication to help us recover, but the timing was not good.

The day of Jim's death, Cindy and Jim's cousin Becky came to our house to give me the terrible news, which I could barely comprehend. Thankfully, Gale was there for me again. His funeral was a few days later in Kentucky, which gave us time to recover from COVID. We were able to make the funeral, see his family and old friends, and give a eulogy, which I really needed to do.

I did not adequately sum up fifty years of great memories, but I did my best. Gale reminded me that some of the best stories Jim and I would tell her were not allowed to be told in church, especially in front of the family. While preparing my thoughts, I was also thinking about the family of the donor who left me his lungs. I felt a lot of remorse, which is taking me a long time to get over.

The grieving takes over from the anger and guilt, but so far neither has fully stopped. However, the sadness is now mixed with great memories and a reminder of my chance to enjoy life so I can make a few more memories. I think Gale is counting on Stan to help keep me out of trouble, just like Jim tried to do (or vice versa).

I quit thinking about what is fair anymore.

While in Florida for Jim's celebration of life, our dog, Colonel, decided it was time to join Jim in heaven. He was the center of our life, and we could not imagine ever having a better companion than him. I have thought warmly about him and Jim every day since.

My transplant evaluation discovered a blockage in the same artery, which is probably what killed Jim. I had a stent that no doubt saved my life. If that does not define life's irony, nothing does.

The celebration of life in Florida was a nice celebration at Jim and Cindy's home in St. Pete Beach, as I spent quality time with his sons, John and Ryan, and his daughter, Heather, plus his seven grandkids. I also met many of the co-workers he had talked about over the years. We all had a good time. Jim had saved a bottle of Rock Hill Farms bourbon for a special occasion. We opened it and passed drinks around that day. My toast was to remind everyone that most days are special and to never allow any dust to accumulate on that special bottle. I also told everyone not to mix it with Coke or he would come back to haunt them.

Jim and I met while attending the University of Kentucky in 1972 at the Chevy Chase Inn over a couple of pitchers of beer. That day we started planning our first fishing trip to Florida and spent many good days on the water together since. We had a lot of adventures over the years. There are no bad days when you are out fishing with your best friend.

Year Two recovery was tough, but I made it. My health had improved, but I was still tired in the afternoons, had several headaches, cataracts, brain fog, joint and muscle pain, and respiratory infections, but I made it to Year Three. I refused to take naps and tried to keep myself moving. While I continued to exercise and ride my bike, I was eating too many doughnuts and desserts and slowly gaining weight. I continued to document in my daily journal about doughnut stops on the way back from lab work at the clinic. There was a new gelato shop that opened on the corner of our street, which I was frequenting way too often. I should have known better.

On my two-year anniversary, I had told Jim I thought I needed to make it through three years with these new lungs in order to get healthy enough to travel. We began planning our next fishing trip adventure right away. We had big plans.

Gale had a business meeting in Scottsdale, Arizona, in late spring 2023. We had previously planned a road trip about the same time to Cottonwood as a base to visit the national parks and all the sights in-between. Her meeting caused us to decide to make a longer trip. Before our trip, Cindy had sent us some photos from Jim's celebration of life, and once I saw those photos of me being overweight, pale, and obviously out of shape, I decided it was time to get things turned around.

While Gale had meetings, I decided to hike to the top of nearby Camelback Mountain. The first day, I was not prepared. I made it about a mile. The second day, I bought better shoes, a hiking stick, and took more water. I was determined to make it to the top or die. It was tough, but I made it.

That was another turning point in my health. We had some great hikes later at the Grand Canyon with Gale's coworkers, and we covered a lot of trails over the next few days. I was stronger when I returned home but still overweight. I reduced my daily intake of doughnuts, desserts, and carbs, and I exercised more. I returned home more determined, then I lost thirty-seven pounds in six months. The only downside was that I had donated most of my outgrown clothes to the Eastern Kentucky flood victims. Now I had to replace them.

This was just a start, but this should set me up for better years ahead while fighting through the bumps in the road I will no doubt have. My ability to read and concentrate is also improving. I realize that the medications I must take will never allow me to get back to where I was, but I believe my greatest barrier to better health is maintaining determination. No one else can *give* you that.

I continue to use my daily journal to track my health progress. I write about my fishing trips and events that Gale and I attend. My anti-rejection medications have been slightly reduced as my labs and exams provide my doctors with data so they can properly tweak my daily pills or shots. If a new vaccine comes out, I am first in line. My transplant clinic trips are now only quarterly unless I have health issues. The side effects must be managed, which requires visits to other specialists.

One friend from our lung transplant support group discovered melanoma a little over a year after his transplant date. The treatments required to balance anti-rejection vs. treatments for fighting cancer are not easy. We spent time together in the rehab clinic and he was a determined fighter. But Larry did not make it. Another friend in our group had terminal complications from COVID. Reality sets in. All lung transplant patients know a complication or rejection can be just a day away. I am reminded of this every time I visit the clinic where I speak to others. In the back of my mind, the reality of life can be mentally taxing at times.

I just spent a day with my old college friends at the Keeneland racetrack. We call ourselves Mae's Kids after my friend Kelly Sinclair's mom, who started our annual get-togethers more than fifty years ago. It was a great day and a true celebration of life and friendship.

This book took a while to finish. I am not sure if getting this far is a miracle or not. I just know I made it further than I expected. My bucket list is waiting. I received the gift of life from my donor, as well as from Gale and my doctors. I am very grateful for this opportunity and the wonderful life I have lived, and for the life I have.

UK Healthcare Article

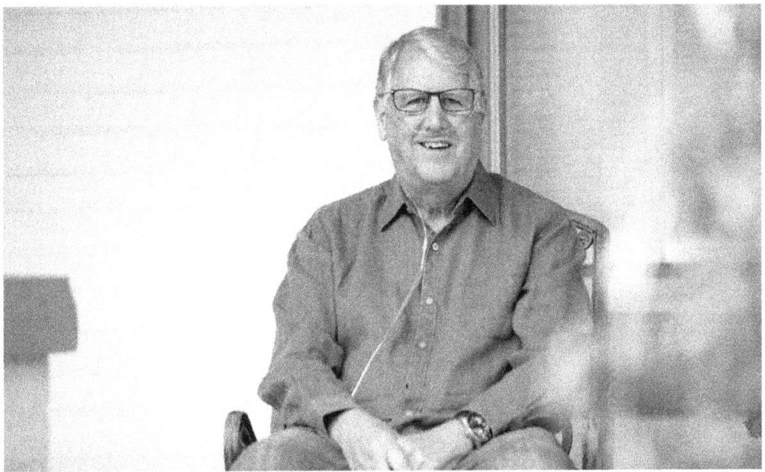

Tom Williams, a UKHC pulmonary fibrosis patient, enjoys a good read on his front porch. Photo by Pete Comparoni | UKphoto

Reprinted with permission by UK HealthCare

LEXINGTON, Ky. (Sept. 25, 2020) — Tom Williams spends his days sitting on the front porch, diving deep into a good book. He has always loved to read but never had enough time to fully enjoy it between busy days at work and home – until now. Now, the front porch is his daily destination. It's the farthest he can leave his Lexington home without compromising his fragile health.

A Kentucky native, Williams was diagnosed with idiopathic pulmonary fibrosis (IPF) in 2018. At the time, he traveled extensively and was living in Houston when he started to experience shortness of breath. Today, he is on life-saving oxygen 20 hours a day and is awaiting a double-lung transplant.

"My life changed rapidly after the diagnosis," Williams said. "You don't realize how fast it changes you. I started keeping a diary and looking back just over a span of three months, I see how it restricted my lifestyle significantly."

More than 200,000 Americans are living with pulmonary fibrosis, a devastating disease that causes progressive scarring in the lungs. Fifty-thousand new cases of PF are diagnosed each year. Idiopathic pulmonary fibrosis, the most common form of the disease, has no known cause and no known cure. The UK Pulmonary, Critical Care and Sleep Medicine Clinic is a part of the Pulmonary Fibrosis Foundation's (PFF) nationwide Care Center Network and the designation allows UK HealthCare to further advance its patients' care by increasing access to treatment and services.

After moving to Lexington for his wife's job, Williams, the former president of a large research organization, plowed into his own research about PF. "I jumped in with gusto," he said. "I did a lot of digging into my family history and connecting with people who I didn't even know were family. In the end, I didn't find anyone on either side of the family who suffered from this disease."

Though there is no way to know for sure, Williams believes it's possible that his lungs suffered significantly from chemicals and dust he breathed during his work in the oil and gas industry decades ago. While masks are mandatory in Kentucky due to COVID-19, Williams urges those who are exposed to hazardous conditions on the job to mask-up even after the coronavirus pandemic is over. "Maybe, had I worn a mask back then when I was around the nasty chemicals and dust, things would have been different for me today," he said.

One critical aspect of Williams' care includes visits to the UK HealthCare Interstitial Lung Disease Clinic. Dr. James McCormick, a specialist in Pulmonary Critical Care and Sleep Medicine and Williams' doctor, said these clinic appointments are necessary to keep patients on track. "Keeping up with our team is vital to helping patients regain the ability to live their normal day-to-day life and restore their independence," McCormick said.

The clinic offers patients with chronic, advanced lung disease the expert care and multidisciplinary resources they need to reduce symptoms, minimize additional damage, and maximize their quality of life.

Williams said the program not only benefited him physically by helping him drop some weight, but it also allowed him to meet others who are fighting the same disease. "You hear their stories and it gives you hope," Williams said. "Most people who go through the transplant process have done very well, so I hope that I have a good chance at a long life on the other side of this."

Waiting for 'the call'

Williams is also now among the nearly 1,000 people in Kentucky waiting for life-saving organs. He has been on the transplant list for 15 weeks. He needs two lungs and is working with UKHC's medical director of Lung Transplant, Dr. Maher Baz, to find a match.

The transplant team at UKHC's Transplant Center performs more than 200 transplant surgeries a year. The center's team of cardiothoracic surgeons, pulmonologists, pharmacists, and nurses works together to determine the appropriate treatment options for each patient, while social workers and support staff help the patients and their families throughout the transplant process—before, during and after surgery.

Hospitals around the world are adapting care around the COVID-19 pandemic, but transplant surgeries and the need for donors is still just as dire. "The coronavirus pandemic has changed the transplant process in some ways, specifically regarding who can receive a transplant and who is eligible to donate," Baz said. "Our team is very thorough in making sure we find the right match that is safe for all involved."

For Williams, this means the only time he leaves his home is to go to the doctor or UK Chandler Hospital for appointments, though some of his appointments are done via UKHC Telehealth.

"If I get COVID, I figure I'm toast," Williams said. "My wife and I have to go to extreme measures to make sure we do everything possible to avoid it. The only time we go out is to the hospital, and of course, we take precautions there to stay safe."

For now, Williams keeps his phone by his side at all times and holds his breath every time it rings. It's a torturous waiting game.

"You never know when you're going to get *the* call that could change everything," he said. "Every time the phone rings, you hope it's 'go-time.' It's very nerve-wracking. The things you do every day are geared around getting that phone call."

In the meantime, Williams sticks to his front porch—and that good book.

Acknowledgments

I learned at an early age that if I wrote something down every day, it was important at the time and would probably be so in the future. This discipline helped me muddle through life fairly well. The older I got, the more it helped supplement my memory. A diary was essential for me in my professional life as well. When I was told I had IPF, I knew my diary would be essential in my recovery. I believed that I would get through this ordeal by documenting the disease and treatment.

The recovery process after an organ transplant is both a physical and mental challenge. I read about this, but I was not sure about the mental part. I figured maybe others would struggle with this, but not me. I was wrong. Reading my diaries was important in my mental recovery. It was not easy because it took me back to events that I'd rather forget. Those memories kept me up many nights. Reading about it made me relive the emotional part of this process, which my mind was trying to suppress, but it was important.

I thought I had a story that may help others. So, I decided to author a book. I have written more than a hundred technical papers and articles about the environment, oil and gas, and research, but a book? In the past, I had co-authors and technical editors who fixed my writings, but this was way different. I reached out to Greg Anderson, whom Rich Haut and I co-authored *Environment 24/7* with in 2012. He gave me the best advice to reach out to Kathleen Pothier, who did an excellent job of editing, especially for taking out all the ramblings that I had initially written from my "less than stellar" state of mind. Then there was Melissa Farr's great graphic design work to put it together. Thank you all.

I finally had my story validated with the two people who got me through this: my wonderful wife, Gale, and my friend Bob Dolence. Thumbs up! With a few fixes, it was ready to go. Writing this did a lot of good for me, and I hope it helps others.

Most importantly, I want to thank everyone who made the decision to donate an organ so others can live.

About the Author

Thomas Williams is a native Kentuckian who spent most of his professional career in the energy business. Growing up in Kentucky, and then later working in Washington, D.C., and Houston, Texas, his professional focus has been on advancing technology to utilize our natural resources in an environmentally responsible manner. He lives in Lexington, Kentucky, with his wife, Gale, where they spend of lot of their free time planning their next adventure.

The net proceeds from this book will go to the Pulmonary Fibrosis Foundation and Donate Life Kentucky.

www.**incurablelungs**.com

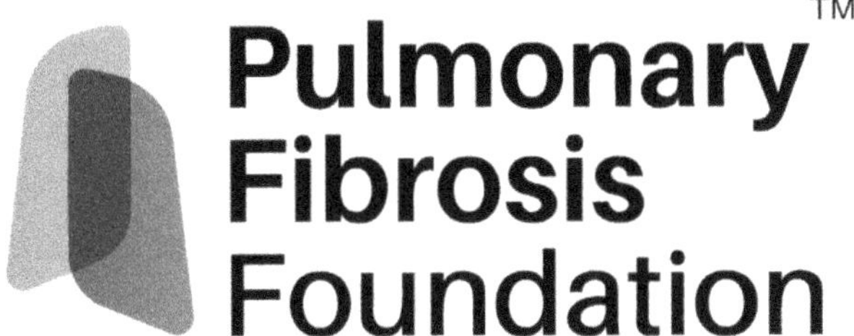

Pulling back the curtain on one's journey with idiopathic pulmonary fibrosis (IPF) is the most effective way to spread awareness of what otherwise is a complex, life-altering disease, with more than 250,000 Americans living with pulmonary fibrosis. Kudos to Tom for selflessly sharing his experience with us. As Tom says, "The more we learn and communicate with others, the better we will all get through it."

The mission of the Pulmonary Fibrosis Foundation is to accelerate the development of new treatments and ultimately a cure. We are committed to advancing improved care of patients and providing unequaled support and educational resources for patients, caregivers, family members, and healthcare providers. To learn more, please visit us at **www.pulmonaryfibrosis.org**.

Your legacy continues when you share your life with others.

Donate Life Kentucky inspires hope through four pillars of support:

- Educates about organ, eye, and tissue donation.
- Ensures that at-risk recipients have access to life-sustaining medical care.
- Grants assistance to children and their families while they await their gift of life.
- Relieves the financial burden that donor families may face after the unexpected loss of their loved one.

Join us by sharing the importance of organ donation with others and make a meaningful financial contribution at **https://bit.ly/DLKYContribute**. Together, let's make a difference and save lives!

www.ingramcontent.com/pod-product-compliance
Ingram Content Group UK Ltd.
Pitfield, Milton Keynes, MK11 3LW, UK
UKHW062308290726
14090UKWH00018B/948

9 798218 507510